THE
SALERNO
SOLUTION

AN OUNCE OF PREVENTION,
A LIFETIME OF HEALTH

DR. JOHN P. SALERNO,

Author of *Fight Fat with Fat*

TAKE
CHARGE
BOOKS

Brevard, North Carolina

Published by Take Charge Books • www.takechargebooks.com
e-mail: TakeChargeBooks2013@gmail.com

The purpose of this book is to educate. It is not intended to serve as a replacement for professional medical advice. Any use of this information in this book is at the reader's discretion. This book is sold with the understanding that neither the publisher nor the authors have any liability or responsibility for any injury caused or alleged to be caused directly or indirectly by the information contained in this book. While every effort has been made to ensure its accuracy, the book's contents should not be construed as medical advice. To obtain medical advice on your individual health needs, please consult a qualified health care practitioner.

Salerno, John.
The Salerno Solution : An Ounce of Prevention, A Lifetime of Health.
Includes bibliographic references and index.

ISBN 978-0-9982658-0-3
Library of Congress Control Number: on file

Editors: Kathleen Barnes and Kate Stockman
Cover and interior design: Gary A. Rosenberg
www.thebookcouple.com

Contents

Introduction

I was lucky to grow up in an Italian family where the dinner table was a place we all gathered to enjoy the family and a meal prepared by my mother and grandmother. Fresh fruits and vegetables, great meat from the corner butcher shop, fish plucked from the sea and pasta my grandmother made with her own two hands was our typical fare. We didn't think anything about this. We thought everybody ate like this. Only as I grew older did I realize that the traditional American diet was far from this fresh food on which I thrived as a child.

I am a part of the Baby Boomer generation, the post-World War II babies who came up in an era when Americans discovered TV dinners, home freezers, canned spaghetti and a host of convenience foods never seen before. In the name of modernity, most Americans gave up good nutrition without even a whimper.

Of course, now we are beginning to reap the harvest of this inadequate diet. Obesity is a national epidemic. Diabetes is rising at an alarming rate. Cancer, heart disease and a host of other diet-related illnesses plague our population.

The conservative American Medical Association has stated that 73 percent of all cancers, stroke and heart disease could be prevented with dietary and other lifestyle modifications. After reviewing the numerous developments in recent medical research, I have become increasingly convinced that the figure is probably closer to 90 percent.

As a holistic family physician, I believe in the body's ability to heal itself. And having had the privilege of practicing with the late, great Dr. Robert C. Atkins, I understand that many of our ills start with poor diet. Fortunately, the corollary is that these same nutrients—in both food and nutritional supplements—can also heal. Dr. Atkins was a pioneer of the low-carb diet and my *Fight Fat with Fat Diet* is a natural outgrowth of Dr. Atkins' work. These diets, which are being validated every day by new research, require strict control of carbohydrate consumption, emphasizing protein and fat as the primary sources of dietary calories in addition to a controlled number of carbohydrates from vegetables.

> Don't wait until you get sick to turn your health around. Be proactive. Then, you can spend your golden years on the tennis court, visiting exotic climes, hiking the Appalachian Trail, building a tree house for your grandchildren or tending a vegetable garden—instead of keeping track of your umpteen prescription drugs, cooling your heels in doctors' offices and subjecting yourself to endless rounds of medical tests.

But can a lifetime of poor nutritional habits be undone?

Ideally, one should start eating healthy in early childhood. But getting off on the wrong foot is no reason to give up. It's never too late to start eating right. I see people in my practice who have been diagnosed with Type 2 diabetes who have reduced or even eliminated their need to take insulin simply by changing the way they eat. This is powerful evidence of the force of nutrition.

I have to refer to my grandfather. He taught me that we should eat "close to the ground," meaning we should consume unprocessed foods as close to the place they were grown as possible. This is easier to do than you might think, even in today's world littered with processed foods. You just have to train yourself to seek the pure and whole foods.

My grandfather lived to be 95. He was seldom sick. I believe that with proper eating habits you, too, can live a long and vigorous life.

In the pages that follow, I'll teach you which foods to eat—and which to leave on the supermarket shelf or buffet table—as well as provide advice on what key nutrients require supplementation.

Of course, it bears repeating that remaining—or becoming—physically fit and minimizing stress are also key to health and longevity.

Introduction to Nutrition

CHAPTER I

Nutrition Basics

Before you eat one bite of food, I'd like to pause a moment for a drink of water.

You are not only what you eat but also what you drink. You won't be surprised to hear that water is the primary liquid you need for good health. You need clean, pure water, the kind you probably won't find coming out of your tap. A solid body of research has also found that two other liquids, namely green tea and red wine, are also health protective.

The source of life

Note that I refer to purified water, not just water. Our toxic environment means it is simply not safe to drink tap water. Why? Municipal water systems have been adulterated with chlorine, fluoride and even a host of prescription drugs. I'll leave it up to your imagination to figure out how Lipitor, Paxil and Viagra, among other commonly used drugs, wound up in the water supplies of many of our major cities.

Nor can you assume that just because water is in a bottle, it is free of contaminants. The only way to be sure the water you consume is free of heavy metals, pesticides and microorganisms like giardia and cryptosporidium is to buy from a certified source or install a quality filtration system yourself.

Drink eight 8-ounce glasses of pure water daily.
Many of us are chronically dehydrated. By the time your
brain tells your body it is thirsty, you are already dehydrated.
Instead of waiting to feel thirsty, start guzzling after breakfast.
One way to get your 64 ounces daily is to fill a quart bottle
every morning and see that you drink it by lunchtime. Do the
same with another quart bottle by dinnertime.

In addition to promoting regularity, lubricating your joints
and helping all your organs function optimally, increasing your
water input automatically increases your urinary output, which
cleanses your body, diluting impurities and eliminating toxins.
Adequate hydration also helps nutrients flow into our cells. If
you are consuming a lot of nutritional supplements, it is even
more crucial that you drink plenty of water.

To your health

Numerous population studies have shown that moderate consumption of alcohol is linked to a decrease in the overall risk of
death from all causes, especially from stroke and cardiovascular
disease. Red wine in particular appears to have additional health
benefits, thanks to its high levels of antioxidants that combat
oxidative stress, which is the cells' degenerative process, acting
much like rust on the bumper of a car. Oxidative stress plays a
role in cancer, coronary artery disease, Alzheimer's disease and
arthritis, among other diseases.

Have a cuppa

Green tea, as well as black and white varieties, also contains
antioxidants to combat the "rust" on aging cells. Green tea is
high in EGCG (epigallocatechins), a compound of four powerful
antioxidants in the catechin family that is more potent than vitamins C and E.

Population studies show that people in cultures where drinking green tea is the norm have lower rates of coronary artery disease. Research has also shown that regularly drinking green tea can lower both total and LDL ("bad") cholesterol, reducing the tendency of blood to clot.

CHAPTER 2

What to Eat
and Where to Find It

Choose unprocessed foods that have been touched as little as possible by agribusiness. This means a fresh chicken, not fried chicken heated in the microwave; fresh green beans, not a frozen vegetable "medley" with a starchy sauce enhanced with chemicals to give it flavor; fresh fruit instead of sugary fruit drinks or baked goods from home or the store. Much of the products that crowd the supermarket shelves are doused with preservatives and other chemicals and may be packed with white flour, sugar and other refined carbohydrates that have seriously negative effects on everyone's health. Focus instead on whole foods.

To get foods with the highest nutrient levels—including the all-important antioxidants—as much as possible seek out *organic* produce and meats which aren't contaminated with chemical fertilizers, pesticides, preservatives and flavor enhancers.

Ideally, choose locally grown produce, perhaps from a farm stand because shipping time is minimal, therefore most of the nutrients have been retained. Ask vendors about their farming methods. You may find that even if a farm is not certified organic (this can take several years), it may be using traditional farming methods rather than chemical fertilizers. When it comes to meat and poultry, avoid any products that use hormones and antibiotics or feed from genetically-modified corn.

A degraded food supply

While a good diet is essential for good health and supplements should never be used in lieu of healthful foods, the quality of much of the food produced in the U.S. today is debased. Food production here has become an industry like manufacturing steel, cars or detergent. While agribusiness has definitely introduced efficiencies and reduced the cost of food relative to income, we have paid a heavy price in terms of quality.

Food is trucked across the country, meaning a head of lettuce picked a week ago has lost much of its nutritional value by the time it reaches your salad bowl. Meat is processed in central locations and then trucked to your supermarket. Increasingly, chemicals and radiation are being used to add shelf life to items that are best consumed immediately after harvest.

Lack of freshness and the ever-present danger of spoilage and possible food poisoning is just the beginning. Dependence on chemical fertilizers to increase output and reduce cost has depleted the soil. Natural farming methods, including crop rotation and enrichment with manure and compost, enable crops to absorb trace minerals and other nutrients from the soil, but fruits and vegetables grown in soil degraded by repeated use of chemical fertilizers contain far fewer nutrients. A study based on U.S. Department of Agriculture data and published in 2004 in the *Journal of the American College of Nutrition* revealed that of the 13 major nutrients found in fruits and vegetables, six have declined substantially over the last 50 years.

Recently grown crops have shown decreases of up to 38 percent in the amount of protein, calcium, vitamin C, phosphorus, iron and riboflavin. According to lead author Donald Davis, Ph.D., of the University of Texas at Austin's Biochemical Institute in the Department of Chemistry and Biochemistry, the situation may be even more dire.

"Perhaps more worrisome would be declines in nutrients we could not study because they were not reported in 1950—magnesium, zinc, vitamin B$_6$, vitamin E and dietary fiber, not to mention phytochemicals," he said.

> Herein lies the double whammy: not only is our air, water and soil increasingly compromised, but our food supply, which would normally enhance our immunity and ability to deal with toxic assaults, lacks the nutrients to protect us. To compound the problem, our diet is increasingly dominated by processed foods without much nutritive value other than calories, especially foods full of white flour, sugar, high fructose corn syrup and other refined carbohydrates.

Most industrialized countries have eliminated hunger as a public health problem, only to have it replaced with another dangerous condition: obesity. And ironically, people who subsist on doughnuts, bagels, cheeseburgers, potato chips, pizza, soft drinks and other junk food may be undernourished and vulnerable to a host of diseases, even though they are well upholstered.

The average American eats only two to three servings of vegetables and fruit a day, missing out on the natural sources for many vitamins and minerals. As you will learn in the chapters that follow, if you are overweight, making dietary changes that result in permanent weight loss is the first thing you can do to improve your health and increase your chances for well-being well into old age. In fact, most of the diseases that plague us in the 21st century that are not linked to our degradation of the environment are associated with excess consumption—specifically heart disease, diabetes and many types of cancer.

CHAPTER 3

Carbs and Veggies and Fruits, Oh My!

My dietary recommendations with my Fight Fat with Fat Diet dovetail well with Dr. Atkins' low-carbohydrate approach, which I have found is effective not just for controlling excess weight but also for preventing disease and correcting health problems.

I know that the Atkins diet erroneously got a reputation of being the "bacon double-cheeseburger diet." My Fight Fat with Fat Diet grew out of my work with Dr. Atkins. It is a three-step proactive approach to nutrition based on:

- organic unprocessed foods,

- high protein, high natural fat and low-carbohydrate, low-glycemic choices,

- approach to nutrition based on fortification with pure organic nutritional supplements targeted to strengthen the immune system, reduce inflammation and destroy free radicals.

It is extremely healthy, as my experience with patients for more than 20 years proves.

The subject of this book is not weight loss, although I hardly need remind you that excess weight is associated with a myriad of health problems. To reduce your risk of disease and maximize your life expectancy, you must get your weight into the normal range. For more detail on the Atkins weight-loss program, known as the induction phase of the Atkins Nutritional Approach, see *The Atkins Essentials* (2004) or *Dr. Atkins' New Diet Revolution* (2002), both published by Avon Books. My book, *Dr. Salerno's Fight Fat with Fat Diet* (Madison Lexington Press, 2010) carries on this work. Essentially, the Atkins diet and the Fight Fat with Fat Diet promote high protein consumption without severe fat limitation and eliminate breads, grains, starchy vegetables and sugar.

Even if you are not carrying extra pounds, if you have elevated blood sugar, the metabolic syndrome, pre-diabetes or full-blown Type 2 diabetes, you need to make dietary changes. The conventional Western diet, high in refined carbohydrates, typically causes the blood sugar level to rise quickly after a meal, stimulating the pancreas to release insulin, which transports the blood sugar to cells from the blood. When the blood sugar level drops too low, it sends out a signal in the form of a craving for more quickly metabolized food—meaning something full of carbohydrates. This vicious cycle leads to overeating and weight gain and can ultimately lead to diabetes if the over-stimulated pancreas becomes less effective at its job and unused muscles become less capable of using the body's natural insulin effectively.

The right carbs

My dietary approach, like that of Dr. Atkins, is not to eliminate carbohydrates, but to eat nutrient- and fiber-rich carbs, such as vegetables, fruit and whole grains and stay away from refined carbohydrates including white bread and rice, baked goods made with refined grains and anything with added sugar or high fructose corn syrup in it.

You have probably heard the term "low glycemic" but may not understand exactly what it means. Basically, the lower the glycemic index (GI) of a food, the less glucose (sugar) it will deliver to your blood stream and therefore the more slowly your blood sugar rises. Not all vegetables are low glycemic: roots, legumes, seeds and starchy vegetables are higher. Most fruits are the middle range; a few, including berries and grapefruit, are relatively low; and a few, like raisins and bananas, are relatively high on the glycemic index and raise blood sugar quickly.

Knowing the glycemic load (GL) of a food is another helpful tool that goes hand-in-hand with the glycemic index. While the glycemic index tells you how quickly a particular food will spike your blood sugar, the glycemic load tells you how much carbohydrate is in each serving. For example, watermelon carries a particularly high GI—72, which puts it right up there with Snickers bars. But because watermelon is largely water and you actually get a relatively small amount of carbohydrate in a serving, its glycemic load is a modest (and healthy) 11. On the other hand, the Snickers bar with a similar GI carries an unhealthful glycemic load of 23. Keeping GI foods below 50 *and* looking for foods with GL of 12 or below will help you make good choices.

You'll find a helpful chart that shows both GI and GL at www.alsearsmd.com/glycemic-index/. Many of you will be happy to learn that a one-ounce Dove dark chocolate bar carries a healthy GI of 23 and a healthy GL of 4.4.

Assuming you are of normal weight—meaning a body mass index (BMI, a measure of your weight relative to your height) of between 20 and 24.9—and you don't have elevated blood sugar, you should be able to eat all or most of the following foods. If your weight stays stable and you feel good, there is no need to count carbohydrates or calories. By the way, BMI is commonly used as an indicator of how fat a person is, but it does not take into account relative proportions of muscle, fat and bone in the body. If you're unsure whether you are overweight (most of us know, if we are really honest with ourselves), check your body fat with one of those commonly available scales that measure it. A fit man should have 14 to 17 percent body fat and a fit woman should have 21 to 24 percent.

- Moderate portions of meat, poultry, fish and tofu

- Moderate portions of cheese and other dairy products

- Eggs (including yolks)

- Olive oil, nut and vegetable oils, butter and other natural fats (not margarine)

- Nuts and seeds

- Salad and other vegetables, but consume potatoes, legumes and other high-glycemic vegetables in moderation

- Berries as well as moderate amounts of low-glycemic fruits; choose whole and avoid juice, which has removed the fiber and concentrated the natural fruit sugars; dried fruits, which concentrate sugars, should be regarded as an occasional treat.

- Whole grains and products made from them, in moderation. Be particularly careful about products containing gluten since gluten levels are extremely high in all modern wheat products. Not only does gluten cause digestive disturbances in some people but also certain substances in gluten cross the blood-brain barrier and trigger the opiate receptors in the brain. Put simply, this means wheat is addictive. Eat a little and you want more. Test yourself to see if you're addicted to wheat by eliminating all gluten products from your diet for a couple of weeks. You might be surprised.

A natural diet

Most of your carbohydrate intake should be in the form of fresh vegetables, which are veritable powerhouses in terms of vitamins and minerals as well as fiber. The old advice to eat a variety of colors of vegetables each day is valid, but be sure to focus primarily on lower glycemic vegetables. For the same reason, don't overdo the fruit.

Eat at least one salad a day and steam, braise or lightly stir-fry—rather than boiling—the rest of your vegetables to retain as many nutrients as possible.

The value of vegetables

Among the reasons it is important to eat a variety of veggies each day is the fact that different groups of vegetables confer different benefits.

Go green. Chlorophyll, found in all green plants, is a potent detoxifier. In addition to spinach and broccoli, sample arugula, asparagus, beet greens, bok choy, collards, dandelion greens, kale and mustard greens.

Not just carrots. Yellow summer squash, pumpkins and other winter squash, sweet potatoes, tomatoes and red and yellow bell peppers are also rich in carotenoids such as beta-carotene, lutein and lycopene, all of which destroy free radicals, enhance immune response and protect cells against ultraviolet (UV) radiation.

Rich in color and nutrients. Purple and red vegetables and fruits such as beets, red and purple grapes, blackberries, strawberries and blueberries contain anthocyanidins, which have both anti-inflammatory and antioxidant properties.

Strong stuff. The group of vegetables known as crucifers are powerful detoxifiers, making them particularly valuable to reduce your risk of developing cancer. The crucifers are the often-maligned vegetables such as broccoli that can be odiferous if overcooked, but are delicious lightly steamed, braised, stir fried or roasted. The cruciferous vegetable family includes arugula, broccoli, Brussels sprouts, cabbage, cauliflower, collard greens, kale, kohlrabi, mustard greens, radishes, rutabaga, turnips, watercress, bok choy and Chinese cabbage, as well as horseradish and wasabi. Make a point of eating a variety of them several times a week—or better yet, daily.

Fruit in moderation

Fruit supplies many of the same nutrients found in vegetables, but it is high in natural sugars and elevates your blood sugar much as refined sugar does. Concentrate on lower-carbohydrate, lower-glycemic choices such as blueberries, strawberries, cherries, cranberries, grapefruit and apples. Avoid fruit juices, which concentrate sugars and eliminate fiber. Avoid dried fruit packed with sugar and chemicals to preserve color and enhance the texture.

More good-for-you foods

Additional foods, beverages and seasonings that should be part of your diet include olive oil, coconut oil, whey and virtually all herbs and spices, especially turmeric and ginger.

The Importance of Fiber

Fiber is well known to scour cholesterol from your system. But fiber also plays a major role in removing toxins—as well as excess estrogen—from the body.

To get your fiber fix, in addition to eating a full complement of low-glycemic vegetables and moderate amounts of low-glycemic fruit—if you are at a healthy weight—you can enjoy whole grains, such as brown rice, oatmeal and buckwheat, and breads made from 100 percent whole grains (if you can tolerate gluten). If you are bothered by constipation, supplement with a tablespoon a day of psyllium husks sprinkled on fruit or in capsule form. A couple of tablespoons of ground flaxseeds are an excellent source of fiber.

VITTLES AND VITAMINS

The chart on the following pages should help you make food choices that ensure you get the nutrients you need while keeping your carb intake under control.

Food	Beta-carotene	Vitamin B₃
Apricots, cantaloupe & peaches	X	
Asparagus*		X
Avocado*		
Beans & legumes		
Beets	X	
Blueberries		
Broccoli*	X	
Cabbage (raw)*		
Carrots**	X	
Cereals & whole grains**		X
Eggs		
Fish**		X
Grapefruit		
Guava		
Kale*	X	
Leafy greens: arugula, spinach, Swiss chard, collard*	X	X
Melons		
Milk		
Mushrooms*		
Nuts**		
Nuts & nut butters**		
Onion*		
Oranges		
Papaya*		
Peppers, all colors, sweet or hot*	X	
Potatoes		
Poultry		X
Pumpkin and other winter squash*	X	
Red meat, especially liver		X
Seeds & seed butters**		
Strawberries		
Sweet peas **	X	
Sweet potato **	X	
Tomatoes*	X	
Vegetable, nut, & seed oils		
Watermelon**		
Wheat germ		
Whole grains**		

* low-glycemic choices   ** Consume in moderation

Vitamin B$_6$	Vitamin C	Vitamin E	Glutathione[†]
			X
			X
X			
	X		
	X		
		X	
X			
X			
	X		
	X		
	X	X	
	X		
			X
X			
		X	
			X
	X		
	X		X
	X		
	X		
	X		
X			
		X	
	X		
	X		
		X	
			X
		X	
		X	

† a powerful antioxidant

CHAPTER 4

The Complex Issues of Fats and Meats

Your body needs fat to sustain life, including building cell membranes and making hemoglobin—which transports oxygen in red blood cells—and producing chemicals that help regulate many of the body's functions. Fats can be divided into three basic types based on their chemical makeup:

- *Saturated fats:* Butter, suet and lard, fats that are usually solid at room temperature and are primarily animal fats; but a few, like palm and coconut oil, come from plants.

- *Monounsaturated fats:* Found in olive oil, nuts and seeds and avocados, are liquid at room temperature.

- *Polyunsaturated fats:* Also liquid at room temperature, are found in corn, canola, safflower, soybean and flaxseed oils, as well as the oil in fatty, cold-water fish.

Although dietary fat is often depicted as a villain, it is vital to understand the differences and the vital functions that each performs. Some, like trans fats (AKA hydrogenated or partially hydrogenated oils), which clog your arteries and have been associated with cancer, are always to be avoided. Others, like the omega-6s found in most vegetable oils, should be consumed in moderation; in contrast, omega-3s offer a host of benefits and olive oil, which is an omega-9, is a prince among oils.

There is general agreement that eating so-called "good" fats such as olive oil and cold-water fish promotes good health. But it is simplistic to associate certain foods with one kind of fat. All natural fats, whether from animals or plants, contain a mix of fatty acids. For example, a broiled hamburger contains 39 percent saturated and 43 percent monounsaturated fat. The important thing is to eat a balance of fats. So, for example, if you're eating red meat or poultry for dinner, be sure to dress your vegetables with olive oil instead of butter and perhaps top your salad with a handful of walnuts.

Essential fatty acids

Essential fatty acids (EFAs) are fats that your body needs but cannot manufacture itself and must therefore get from food or dietary supplements. Found in polyunsaturated fats, EFAs include omega-3 fatty acids (or alpha linolenic acids, ALA) and omega-6 fatty acids (or gamma linoleic acids, GLA). Good sources of omega-3s include flaxseeds and flaxseed oil, pumpkin seeds and walnuts. Other forms of omega-3 EFAs are eicosapentaenoic acid (EPA) and docosahexaenoic acid (DHA), found in cold-water fish such as salmon, cod, trout, Atlantic mackerel and sardines, eggs and dark leafy green vegetables, as well as in fish oil supplements and blue-green algae supplements.

Trans fats

Trans fats are manufactured, chemically altered fats like those found in many peanut butters, baked goods and fast food French fries, among others. Eating these abominations in the form of hydrogenated or partially hydrogenated oils found in most margarines and many other processed foods hits your body with a triple whammy: they elevate bad LDL and triglyceride levels and reduce good HDL levels. In a scientific study, subjects ate a comparison diet in which the fat came from butter, a saturated fat without any trans fats. Interestingly, although butter produced the highest cholesterol levels, it also provided the highest proportion of "good" large, fluffy LDL particles (an explanation of fluffy LDL is explained on page 44).

The meat of the matter

Many nutritionists and physicians indict the consumption of red meat as a risk factor for cancer and cardiovascular disease because of its saturated fat content. To be sure, a number of studies have concluded that eating meat is bad for your health.

But I beg to differ, both from my clinical observations and because there are several huge flaws in all these studies.

As a practitioner who worked at the side of Dr. Robert C. Atkins and who prescribes a low-carbohydrate, low-glycemic dietary approach for most of my patients, my experience is completely at odds with this assumption. Many of Dr. Atkins' patients, some who had been with him for up to 20 years, are now my patients. This means that I have medical records on people who have been eating a high-protein diet for up to 30 years. Only a fraction of them have developed cancer in any form.

When it comes to the research, there are at least four reasons why studies on meat consumption are flawed.

1. More of the fat in red meat is monounsaturated or polyunsaturated than saturated. According to the USDA nutrient analysis database, a 3-ounce broiled hamburger patty (85 percent lean) has 5 grams of saturated fat, 5.7 grams of monounsaturated fat and 0.4 grams of polyunsaturated fat. Remember that monounsaturated oils like olive oil are considered health protective.

The meat that 99.9 percent of the population eats is not organic, meaning the animals were pumped full of hormones to increase their weight, given prophylactic antibiotics to prevent disease in cramped conditions and fed grain treated with hormone-disrupting pesticides. Unless studies looked at the effect over years of conventionally farmed meat compared to organic meat, there is no way to ascertain what effect, if any, was inherent in the meat itself or the hormones, antibiotics or pesticides in combination or as individual factors. By the way, all of these toxins settle in the animal's fat, which could be an argument for eating low fat meats if you can't afford organic.

2. Nor did the studies distinguish between people who ate both red meat and "bad" carbohydrates such as baked goods made with flour and sugary junk foods and those who ate meat and only "good" carbohydrates like vegetables and whole grains. The combination of a high fat and a high carbohydrate diet—epitomized by Americans' favorite meal of a burger and French fries, probably cooked with carcinogenic partially hydrogenated oils—is a recipe for disaster.

3. Finally, these studies do not distinguish between those who eat their hamburgers and lamb chops medium rare and those who prefer them well done. Charred meat is a known carcinogen. How can we tell whether the meat itself was to blame in population studies without designing the study to make a distinction between the two? It's also important to note that eating rare grass-fed beef carries with it a substantially lower risk of bacterial contamination than with beef from cattle fed antibiotics and hormones.

I advocate eating many forms of protein, not just red meat. There is nothing wrong with organically raised beef and other red meat, but if you eat steak to the exclusion of pork, poultry, fish, eggs, cheese and soy products, you're missing out on their health benefits. There may be some hormonal risks from certain types of soy products, but in general fermented soy is fine.

What about kids?

Parents and caregivers play a key role in making healthy choices for children and in teaching children to make healthy choices for themselves. It can be a challenge to get kids to eat well. But with today's skyrocketing numbers of kids who have obesity and diabetic issues, it is mandatory that they are educated about and offered healthy foods. Making these changes can set your kids on the road to better health. Although adults usually decide what kids eat, we all know that kids eat what is available. Therefore, surrounding them with healthier options leaves them no choice but to eat better food. This isn't rocket science. But it isn't easy: it takes attention and planning. Here are a few suggestions:

- First, if you are new to parenthood, breast milk is one of the most effective obesity prevention tools, and breastfeeding is an excellent way to get your baby started on living a nutritious life.

- Serve kids fresh, frozen, and canned fruits and vegetables; they all count.

- Offer whole fruit or 100 percent juice, with no added sugar.

- Mix vegetables into dishes, like adding peas to rice, or cucumbers to a sandwich.

- Use whole fat milk, yogurt and cheese.

- Choose good quality cuts of meat like skinless chicken or extra lean ground beef for hamburgers or pasta sauces.

- Bake or grill instead of fry.

- Choose high quality olive oil or butter.

- Substitute water or milk for sodas or sweetened beverages.

- Eliminate soda or sugar-sweetened drinks.

- Switch to low-sugar breakfast cereals.

- Switch to fruit-based desserts.

- Reduce the number of snacks served each day.

- Differentiate between snacks that require permission (cookies), versus snacks that kids can take freely (fresh or dried fruit)

- Provide fruit or carrot sticks as great snacks.

- Have kids drink water at snack time.

- Kids are smaller than adults and should eat smaller portions.

- Use smaller plates for kids.

- Don't force kids to clean their plates if they are full.

- Portions should be about the size of the back of a fist (a child's fist for a child's portion).

- Start with a small portion. Children can have seconds if they are still hungry.

- For older children, there is a popular slogan to help kids learn how to be healthy. It goes "5-2-1-almost none." This is a slogan to learn and take to heart. Five is for eating five servings of fruits and vegetables every day. Two is for no more than two hours of screen time per day (nonschool related and does include cell phone time). One is for at least one hour of exercise each day, and "almost none" is for the amount of sugar-sweetened drinks you and your kids should drink (includes sodas, sports drinks, and sweet tea). Just eliminating one soda per day equals losing almost 15 pounds in a year.

- Planning meals ahead can help. Having fruits and vegetables on hand can help. Try keeping some oranges or apples in a bowl in the kitchen. When hungry kids come home and that is what they find, you might be surprised to see them munching on a piece of fruit.

- Another trick to improve nutrition is to make sure you and your kids eat breakfast every day. Grab a yogurt or granola bar on the way out the door if you don't have time to sit down.

- Drink lots of water. This is good for your health in so many ways, but most importantly helps you maintain a healthy weight. Most of us do not get enough water, but with kids carrying around water bottles at school now, this might be changing.

- Other ways to help your family eat better include making a pledge to remove electronics from mealtime. That means turning off the TV and putting away cell phones. Studies show that people eat more when eating in front of the TV.

- Eating more meals at home is great for family conversation and results in eating less. Eating out often makes us double and triple portion sizes. A little trick is that the size of your meat should equal the size of your fist.

- Slow down mealtime and eat dinner in courses starting with the fruits and vegetables.

- Regularly scheduled meal and snack times help kids learn structure for eating. Eating together is a chance to model good behavior. Focus on eating and enjoying food and each other.

Finally . . . here's a bit more contrarian thinking. I love bacon and I think it's healthy.

BaconFreak.com is the ultimate online Bacon superstore. They sell three dozen varieties of gourmet bacon, including nine different varieties of nitrate-free bacon. Their "Bacon of the Month Club" includes automatic monthly deliveries of their thick-cut, artisan bacon to their customers' doors. The "Bacon of the Month Club" is available in a nitrate-free version. They were also the first company to create Bacon Jerky.

Their blog, BaconToday.com, attracts a wide range of readers, both men and women, who are interested in their bacon recipes and the latest bacon news. Their blog features many original recipes utilizing bacon as a key ingredient. Their products have been featured in *People, Maxim, Sports Illustrated, The Wall Street Journal, Comfort Food, 805 Living, Glamour,* and *Inc.* Magazines. They've also been featured on many TV shows including Destination America's *United States of Bacon* and the Travel Channel's *Food Paradise.*

CHAPTER 5

The Salerno Solution Basic Supplement Program

No matter how focused you are on a healthy diet, it is almost impossible to get all the nutrients you need in the right proportions. The loss of nutrients in fruits and vegetables during transport and even the declining soil quality may leave any of us lacking.

I'm adding here a short list of general supplements that almost everyone should take on a daily basis. You'll see in subsequent sections recommendations for other supplements that address specific risks, like heart disease, diabetes and cancers.

Multi-vitamin

Take a good quality multi-vitamin every day. I think of it as an insurance policy. I recommend whole food organic multi-vitamins that concentrate the entire nutrient molecules. Most non-organic multi-vitamins contain synthesized products that call themselves molecules of vitamins (as in vitamin A, which almost always is typified as beta-carotene, while, in fact vitamin A and all other vitamins, have a dozen or more other essential nutrients that must work with each other).

Optimal daily dose: Take according to manufacturer's instructions.

Fish oil

You'll need a good quality fish oil supplement unless you're eating wild caught cold-water fish three times a week. Look for a product that is certified as free of heavy metals. Krill, tiny fish that are at the bottom of the food chain and therefore less likely to have concentrated mercury and other heavy metals in their flesh, are a good choice. Fish oil has two main ingredients, EPA and DHA. Look for a product that guarantees a total of one gram of the two combined each day. If the fishy burp revolts you, look for enteric-coated capsules that don't dissolve until they are ready to leave your stomach.

Optimal daily dose: A minimum of 250 mg of EPA and 500 mg of DHA

Minerals

Minerals are essential to all functions of the body, but unbalanced intake of minerals (such as taking large amounts of calcium without others to balance it) can cause serious health problems. Look for an ionic trace mineral supplement made from sea salt to give you absorbable amounts of those esoteric trace minerals that are so important to optimal body function. You can find them in liquid and capsule forms.

Optimal daily dose: According to manufacturer's instructions

Vitamin C

We humans cannot produce this essential vitamin ourselves; instead, we must get it from food and supplements. More than 40 percent of Americans don't get even 60 mgs a day—the current RDA is 75 mg for women and 90 for men. However, the RDA is based upon preventing deficiency, not promoting optimal health. Most of us need much more vitamin C than these minimal amounts.

Extensive research on vitamin C has confirmed its heart protective capability as well as its abilities to help build strong blood vessels, connective tissues and other soft tissues.

Optimal daily dose: 500–3,000 mg of Ester-C or a whole food vitamin C

CHART OF BASIC SUPPLEMENTS

More detailed information is available starting on page 27. Those with * have cautionary notes in the text.

SUPPLEMENT			BENEFITS		
	General Health	Heart Disease[†]	Diabetes	Cancers	Alzheimer's[†]
Multi-vitamin	X			X	
Vitamin C	X	X	X		X
Vitamin D	X		X	X	X
Vitamin E*	X	X			
Minerals	X	X	X		
Turmeric/Curcumin		X	X	X	
Fish Oil (Omega-3)*	X	X	X	X	X
Coenzyme Q10*	X	X	X	X	X

[†] and related disorders

Vitamin D

Current research is showing us such remarkable effects of vitamin D that range from prevention of cancer, heart disease, osteoporosis, diabetes and more as well as strengthening immune function. However, most of us are deficient in vitamin D, especially in winter, because our bodies manufacture it from skin exposure to the sun. By all means get yourself a simple blood test to determine your levels, but most of us need a supplement.

Optimal daily dose: 1,000 to 5,000 IU of vitamin D3 in winter, less if you regularly expose most of your skin to strong sunlight.

Coenzyme Q-10

The fat-soluble antioxidant Coenzyme Q-10 (Co Q-10) is a compound found in the mitochondria, or energy center, of every cell of the body, with the greatest concentration in the heart, which, in part, helps it to pump forcefully. As an antioxidant, Co Q-10 also scavenges free radicals. It also inhibits the formation of clots.

Extreme deficiency of Co Q-10 can lead to impaired energy production, oxidative stress and heart failure. It's especially important for people taking statin drugs to take Co Q-10 because the drugs deplete the body's stores of the nutrient.

Optimal daily dose: 100–200 mg

In Conclusion

You are what you eat. A healthy diet will serve you well, prevent disease and help you to live a long, vibrant life. If I could put all of the advice in this a chapter into a nutshell, I'd say:

- Eat a low-carb diet.

- Avoid processed foods, sugar, trans fats and refined grains.

- Choose organic vegetables, fruits and meats as much as you can.

- Train your kids to eat well from childhood into adulthood to give them the best chance at a lifetime of health.

Preventing Heart Disease, Stroke and Hypertension

Mr. G came to me eight years ago for weight loss and overall health improvement. He told me to me that his dad died at the age of 51 from an acute heart attack. His brother died of a stroke at 43 and his dad's brother also died of a stroke at 51. His mom and her brother also had heart attacks in their fifties, but survived. Mr. G was a walking time bomb and he was 70 pounds overweight.

His insulin and glucose levels were extremely high as were his homocysteine levels, fibrinogen, lipid protein, triglycerides, cholesterol and oxidized LDL—all strong and independent predictions of heart disease and stroke. As an enthusiastic fish eater, Mr. G's mercury levels were also extremely high, another strong independent risk factor of heart disease. Mr. G was also quite sedentary as a lawyer for a big New York City firm and ate whatever he wanted. His blood antioxidant levels were also very low. Much needed to be done for Mr. G to prevent the same fate as his dad, brother and uncle.

Mr. G was given weekly chelation intravenous therapies to treat his mercury toxicity and placed on my strong multi-vitamin, mineral and antioxidant formula. He was also given a natural formula to lower his homocysteine levels, my glucose formula to lower his insulin and blood glucose, plenty of my mercury-free formula to lower triglycerides, cholesterol and fibrinogen—which also allows blood to flow more freely. Mr. G was encouraged. He hired a personal trainer and practiced yoga and meditation and started on a severely restricted low-carb organic diet for one year, a diet much lower in fat than he would have liked.

To his amazement after that year, Mr. G's blood panels all normalized. He felt great, his body weight was normal; he was free of mercury and essentially risk-free for the heart disease and stroke that have plagued his family.

The trio of cardiovascular diseases—heart disease, stroke and hypertension—is by far the leading cause of death in the U.S., accounting for one of every 2.7 deaths. The tragedy is that many of those deaths were preventable, if the patients had been non-smokers, normalized their weight, been physically active and made other simple lifestyle changes. In this chapter, you'll learn how to dramatically reduce your chances of sharing their fate.

Heart disease, stroke and hypertension all involve the vascular system and are, to a large extent, entwined. All are caused or aggravated by many of the same risk factors and all of them can be kept at bay with positive lifestyle choices.

Arteries and veins carry oxygenated blood from your heart and return oxygen-depleted blood to your heart as well as the entire network of tiny arteries and capillaries, which make up your vascular system. This, in turn, is part of the circulatory system, which also includes the fist-sized muscle that is your heart—constantly expanding and contracting as it pumps blood in and out—and your lungs, which oxygenate your blood. As it makes its long round trip, blood reaches every cell in your body—including your brain—delivering oxygen and nutrients and collecting waste products and carbon dioxide. The job of the liver and kidneys is to clean the blood of these wastes.

According to American Heart Association, more than 71 million Americans had one or more forms of cardiovascular disease (CVD). This figure includes coronary artery disease (CAD), stroke and high blood pressure, as well as myocardial infarction, meaning an acute heart attack, and angina pectoris, chest pain resulting from decreased blood flow to the heart.

CHAPTER 6

The Complex Relationship Within the Trio of Cardiovascular Diseases

There are many forms of heart disease, but I will focus on coronary artery disease, which is the most common—more than 13 million Americans suffer from it, about 6 million of whom are women. It is also the leading cause of death in the U. S., accounting for one in five deaths, for a total of more than 500,000 deaths each year.

Coronary artery disease (CAD), which is also called coronary heart disease (CHD), is caused by a condition called atherosclerosis or hardening of the arteries, which keeps blood from flowing freely to the heart, starving it of oxygen. Atherosclerosis can cause many heart problems including angina pectoris, which affects about 6.5 million Americans, and/or results in one of the 1.2 million acute heart attacks and nearly 800,000 strokes that occur in this country each year.

Atherosclerosis occurs when the arteries that supply blood to the heart become hardened and narrowed with plaque, which is the buildup of cholesterol, triglycerides (a form of fat), calcium and other substances in the blood deposited on the artery walls. There is evidence that atherosclerosis is initiated by damage to the innermost lining of the arteries, called the endothelium, which first allows these substances to collect on the artery walls. This buildup, in turn, stimulates cells in the artery walls to produce other substances that combine to create larger plaques that further thicken the endothelium, reducing the size of the passage through which blood flows.

High blood pressure also plays a role in increasing the risk of atherosclerosis. Tobacco smoke worsens the condition as well and speeds its spread throughout the blood vessels in the entire body.

If plaque in the arteries ruptures, a clot (thrombus) can result. If the clot blocks the artery, it can completely cut off the flow of blood and the supply of oxygen. If the clot breaks off and is carried through the vascular system to another part of the body, it is called an embolus. A heart attack is the result of a clot blocking an artery to the heart, while most strokes are caused by blockage in a vessel that goes to the brain.

Stroke

According to the Centers for Disease Control and Prevention, each year about 800,000 people experience a new or recurrent stroke. About 130,000 people die of strokes and nearly half of all Americans are at risk of stroke. When considered separately from other cardiovascular diseases, stroke ranks number four among all causes of death, behind heart disease, cancer and chronic respiratory disease.

Strokes can vary in severity, but just a few minutes of oxygen deprivation can kill brain cells, so the effects of a stroke can be permanent and include a myriad of symptoms. On the short list are paralysis, weakness on one side of the body and loss of the ability to speak.

Although a stroke can also be caused by a fall or other trauma, I will confine my discussion of strokes to the two types caused by blood clots and other particles that block an artery. Most such strokes are either a cerebral thrombosis or a cerebral embolism, both of which block blood flow to the brain. The former is the more common and occurs in an atherosclerotic artery that feeds the brain. In the latter, a clot traveling through the

bloodstream lodges in an artery in or near the brain. Hemorrhagic strokes, caused by ruptured blood vessels in the brain,
account for about one-fourth of all strokes.

Hypertension

Hypertension, the medical term for high blood pressure, is
called the silent killer. It is estimated that 65 million Americans—
one-third of all adults—have this condition, although about one-
third of those are unaware that they have it. The 26,634 deaths
attributed to the disease in the U.S. in 2010 vastly understate the
seriousness of hypertension because it is a factor in many other
potentially fatal diseases and conditions, including diabetes and
kidney failure as well as heart failure, heart attack and stroke. It
also can negatively impact cognitive functioning.

Although some abnormalities can cause high blood pressure,
most of the time the cause of hypertension is unknown. Healthy
arteries are flexible, able to stretch and contract easily in
response to 60 to 80 heartbeats per minute. As blood pumps
through your arteries, it exerts pressure against the artery walls,
prompting them to dilate or contract in response to the heart's
rhythm. Dilation allows the blood to move through easily, while
contracting restricts blood flow and increases pressure inside the
vessels. Blood pressure rises with each beat of the heart and falls
with each interval when the heart muscle relaxes.

Chronic high blood pressure strains your heart by making it
pump harder. It can damage blood vessels as well as the kidneys
and brain, although all these organs and vessels can deal with
the pressure without *apparent* ill effects for a long time. When
high blood pressure is paired with being overweight and/or having high cholesterol or diabetes, the risk of stroke and heart
attack increases dramatically.

Sleep, exercise and other factors effect blood pressure, so readings fall within a range, rather than remaining fixed. Two numbers comprise your blood pressure, which is portrayed as a ratio.

The top number (which is always higher) is your systolic pressure, measured while the heart beats; the bottom number is your diastolic pressure, and is lower because it measures when your heart is at rest between beats. Ideally, an adult's blood pressure should be less than 120/80, stated as 120 over 80. Numbers above these are considered hypertension. If you are consistently in the range of 120 to 139/80 to 89, you have what is called pre-hypertension.

It is important for you to know your blood pressure level. Your health care provider most likely checks it at each visit, but it is a good idea to get in the habit of taking it yourself with a home kit. Recently, researchers found that taking your blood pressure at home yields more accurate results than the ones you'd generate at the doctor's office. (The idea is that you're calmer at home.) However, a new study published in *The American Journal of Cardiology* found you might not want to completely rely on automatic blood pressure monitors' results. Researchers from the University of Southern California found some startling discrepancies between the newer automatic blood pressure readers and the more traditional mercury manometer/stethoscope combo. The automatic monitors consistently produced lower results, meaning you could have high blood pressure, or pre-hypertension, and think your health is not at risk. A doctor's equipment may give the most accurate BP measurement, but you can bring in your home machine for comparison.

CHAPTER 7

Assessing Your Risks

The litany of risk factors for cardiovascular disease should be all too familiar to you. For the most part, they are the same for most other diseases: aging, being overweight, not exercising regularly, having a high level of stress, smoking, and of course, abusing alcohol or cocaine. Since cholesterol buildup has been seen in children, it's important to assess risk factors and take preventive measures even at the age of five or six.

Factors within your control

I'll dispense with the last one quickly, because it is obvious. Many people who die from cocaine usually succumb from the drug's impact on the heart, including heart attacks and strokes.

High blood pressure is itself an independent risk factor for heart disease and stroke. Individuals over the age of 40 double their risk of heart disease and stroke for each 20/10 points over 115/75. New research also links the infection and inflammation of gums, teeth and the bones that support them with an increased risk for CAD. One study showed that heart patients were significantly more likely to have periodontitis (gum disease) than people without heart disease. People with gum disease were also more likely to experience a heart attack or stroke.

When it comes to heart health, cardiovascular risk and hormone replacement therapy (HRT), it's important to know the differences between bioidentical and synthetic hormones. While bioidentical hormones can actually improve your heart health, synthetic hormones may increase your risk of cardiovascular problems. The most recent research indicates that women who take *synthetic* HRT to relieve symptoms of menopause increase their risk of blood clots, heart attack and stroke. Unlike bioidentical hormones, synthetic hormones are not molecularly identical to the hormones your body naturally produces, so the body recognizes them as foreign.

Additionally, having high cholesterol and eating saturated fat are often cited as risk factors for cardiovascular disease, but as you will soon see, both are oversimplifications of much more complex issues.

Factors beyond your control

Despite the common assumption that you are at elevated risk for heart disease if one of your parents had cardiovascular disease, there is little research that supports this theory. One exception is having a parent who developed early-onset CAD, meaning before age 55.

There also is a gene for a certain lipoprotein, known as apolipoprotein E4, which comes in several forms. People who inherit one of these versions of the gene from both parents are likely to develop familial hypercholesterolemia, which causes very high cholesterol levels and an increased risk for CAD, heart attack and stroke.

People with both Type 1 and Type 2 diabetes are also far more likely to develop CAD and two-and-a-half times more likely to have a stroke than other people.

Age and gender

Along with the rest of your body, your blood vessels become less flexible over the years, making your arteries more susceptible to atherosclerosis and hypertension. Incidence and death rate for all forms of cardiovascular disease rise significantly with age. Men's risk for CAD begins to inch upward at age 45, while women have a 10-year grace period before they face similar increases. The likelihood of being hypertensive increases with every decade. After age 75, more than 70 percent of American men and almost 85 percent of women have high blood pressure. Blood pressure should be kept at normal to avoid these risks. There are many ways to accomplish this, and the last resort should be pharmaceuticals.

Because women live longer than men, more women than men die of stroke each year. Women account for about 60 percent of U.S. stroke deaths.

Although cardiovascular disease clearly is associated with age, research has shown that the process of plaque buildup in the arteries begins in childhood. This makes it especially important to create and nurture good eating habits even in young children.

Racial inequality

African Americans are significantly more at risk for CAD, hypertension and stroke than Caucasians. African Americans are two to three times more likely to have a stroke and to die from one than are whites. Native Americans, Hispanic Americans, native Hawaiians and some Asian Americans also have a higher risk factor for all cardiovascular disease. People of these ethnicities may be at higher risk because of genetics, but also because of poor diet, a sedentary lifestyle, socioeconomic shortfalls and lack of access to preventive medical care.

Lifestyle choices

Two major population studies conducted by researchers at the Harvard School of Public Health underscore the importance of lifestyle choices in preventing cardiovascular diseases. One looked at the impact of lifestyle factors such as diet, exercise, body mass index and smoking on the likelihood of developing

CAD. Almost 43,000 men aged 40 to 75 years were monitored for 16 years as part of the Health Professionals Follow-up Study. Based on answers to questionnaires, men were considered at low risk if they didn't smoke, were of normal weight, exercised for half an hour a day, were moderate drinkers and ate a diet in compliance with government guidelines. At the end of the study, more than 2,000 men had developed CAD, but those with the low-risk lifestyle were 87 percent less likely to have it than those categorized as having a high-risk lifestyle.

The other study followed almost 38,000 healthy women aged 45 and older for roughly a decade and found that those who lived the healthiest lifestyles had 55 percent lower chance of suffering a stroke than those with the least healthy lifestyles.

Both studies make it clear that most cardiovascular disease is preventable. The study on CAD further emphasizes that it is not too late to make changes in midlife or later to lower one's risks.

Get rid of excess weight

Being overweight is usually the result of a combination of poor dietary choices and overeating and a "couch potato" lifestyle. Genes, metabolic disorders and even certain drugs can also play a role. Regardless of the reason(s), if you are overweight (meaning a body mass index, or BMI, of 25 to 29.9) or clinically obese (a BMI of 30 or greater), your chances of developing CAD, stroke or hypertension—as well as many other diseases—are significantly increased. By itself, obesity is an independent risk factor for cardiovascular disease. Excess pounds also increase the likelihood you will engage in other risky lifestyle choices, including lack of exercise and a diet high in sugar, simple carbohydrates and processed foods.

Increasingly scientists have come to understand that fat tissue doesn't just sit there. Rather, it is metabolically active, producing and releasing substances into the bloodstream that help cause other risk factors for CVD such as atherosclerosis, hypertension, inflammation and glucose intolerance. Obesity is also associated with blood vessel constriction that could cause hypertension.

Apples vs. pears

The distribution of fat is also significant. Apple-shaped people carry their weight around the waist and are far more prone to cardiovascular disease than those whose weight settles in their thighs and buttocks, giving them more of a pear shape.

A study of more than 170,000 people in 63 countries confirms that waist size alone is the single best indicator of risk for cardiovascular disease, more so than the amount of fat. For women, this generally means that a waist of more than 35 inches increases risk. For men, the number is 40 inches.

The role of cholesterol

Until a few decades ago, cholesterol was considered bad—end of discussion. Now there is a more nuanced understanding of the role it plays in the body as well as the distinctions among different types of cholesterol. Finally, the role of cholesterol in forming plaque that causes atherosclerosis turns out to be far more complex than originally thought. Let me untangle this complicated subject as briefly and simply as possible.

What is cholesterol?

Let's first deal with some misconceptions.

- Cholesterol is not a fat. Rather, it's a waxy substance that can be transported by fats (lipids) in your blood stream.

- Cholesterol is essential for forming cell membranes, brain tissue, and many hormones—including sex hormones—and insulating your nerve cells. A total cholesterol level below 160 mg/dL is associated with a higher risk of premature death from stroke, cancer and respiratory illness. Your body needs cholesterol to produce vitamin D and to make bile, which is essential to digestion and elimination. Eating a low-fat diet alone won't significantly cut your cholesterol because your liver produces most of it; just a small amount of cholesterol comes from animal foods and your body absorbs only a small percentage of that.

• Some types of cholesterol are good for you and others are bad.

To state it boldly: Without cholesterol, you would die.

In order for the waxy cholesterol to travel in watery blood, the liver coats it with protein. Lipids are fats, waxes and steroids, which is why scientists use the term lipoprotein, meaning a mixture of cholesterol and protein, to refer to the cholesterol in your blood.

There are a number of lipoproteins, but the two most important are:

1. *Low-density lipoprotein* (or LDL) cholesterol carries cholesterol *from* the liver to the parts of the body that need it. It is simplistically called "bad" cholesterol, because high blood levels of it are associated with an increased risk of heart disease.

2. *High-density lipoprotein* (or HDL) cholesterol called "good" cholesterol, removes cholesterol from your blood and other storage sites before it can oxidize and damage blood vessels. HDL cholesterol protects your body by returning cholesterol *to* the liver, which turns most of it into bile so it can be excreted. People with high HDL have a lower risk of heart disease.

The higher your HDL and the lower your LDL, the better. According to the National Cholesterol Education Program (NCEP III), your total cholesterol, which combines LDL and HDL, should be less than 200 mg/dL, and your LDL should be less than 100 to 130 mg/dL. Men should have HDL of at least 40 mg/dL; a woman's should be at least 50 mg/dL. Higher readings of LDL and lower readings of HDL increase your risk of CAD and stroke.

The particulars of particles

Now that you understand about "good" and "bad" cholesterol, I'm afraid I have to throw a wrench into the works. Both HDL and LDL cholesterol are composed of particles of different sizes and densities. Very low-density lipoprotein (VLDL) particles are relatively large and fluffy, compared to intermediate-density lipoprotein (IDL). Low-density lipoprotein (LDL), made up of small, dense particles is most apt to stick to your artery walls, causing atherosclerosis. So a high LDL level might not be that dangerous if you have primarily the light, fluffy Type A LDL. On the other hand, having a high proportion of small, desnse and sticky Type B increases your risk of heart disease. Research has shown that men with CAD have a higher proportion of these small, dense and sticky Type B particles.

Particle size may also help identify individuals who are at heightened risk for CAD. A retrospective study that used data from the Harvard-based Physicians Health Study, which followed almost 15,000 male doctors for several years, linked small LDL particle size in apparently healthy men to a greater likelihood of having a heart attack. When they were divided into five groups by particle size, men with the smallest, densest LDL particles Type B were more than three times more likely to have a heart attack than those with the largest, fluffiest Type A particles. It is estimated that about 25 to 35 percent of healthy men and about 40 to 50 percent of men with heart disease have Type B particles. High levels of Type B are also associated with other cardiovascular risk factors, including low levels of HDL ("good") cholesterol, elevated triglycerides (see below) and insulin resistance.

I always test my patients for Type B as well as for their total

HDL and LDL cholesterol levels. Likewise, I look at the level of lipoprotein, known as lipoprotein(a). A high level of lipoprotein(a) is an independent risk factor for cardiovascular disease. Your total cholesterol to HDL ratio should be 4.5 or under. For example, if your HDL is 60 and your total cholesterol is 140, then your HDL ratio is 2.5. That said, contrary to popular opinion, the opinions of many of my colleagues and the intensive advertising that bombards us daily, cholesterol is really not a major player in CAD risk.

Triglycerides and more

Your level of another blood lipid is also a measure of your risk for cardiovascular disease. Eating too much sugar and/or refined carbohydrates raises triglycerides, the fat globules in your blood. It has become increasingly clear that it is the ratio of HDL to triglycerides, not high total cholesterol, which puts you at heightened danger for atherosclerosis and thus cardiovascular disease. The combination of high LDL, low HDL and high triglycerides is a particularly dangerous combination. So reducing LDL cholesterol may not really decrease your risk for developing cardiovascular disease if you don't also address high triglycerides.

According to the American Heart Association, your triglyceride level should be 150 mg/dL or less. Anything above that figure increases your risk for heart disease. Most of the drugs that address cholesterol levels have no impact on triglycerides, but as you will read, you can reduce high triglycerides with diet and nutritional supplements.

In addition to cholesterol and triglycerides, other blood markers are also indicators of cardiovascular problems:

- *C-reactive protein (CRP)* is a marker for inflammation. Levels of CRP rise when blood vessels are inflamed, which may play an important role in the development of atherosclerosis. An elevated blood level of CRP can signal that you are at risk for CAD.

- *Fibrinogen* is a clotting factor. High blood level of fibrinogen is another independent risk factor for CAD.

- *Homocysteine* is an amino acid produced by the body when the intake of certain vitamins, including B vitamins, is low. Elevated levels of homocysteine have been linked to damage to blood vessel walls, increased risk of premature CAD and blood clots from atherosclerosis, even in people with healthy cholesterol levels.

Triglyceride, homocysteine and CRP levels can be controlled with diet and supplements.

The role of the environment

Scientists studying human genetics are increasingly coming to the conclusion that variations in certain environmentally responsive genes can make us more susceptible to certain diseases, including cardiovascular disease.

It may well be that what have been considered genetic or racial predispositions to certain diseases are more the result of responses to environmental factors. This could explain, for example, why black Nigerians are far less apt to have hypertension than African Americans.

It will be decades, if ever, before the genetic and environmental factors that cause diseases are untangled. Meanwhile, we do know plenty about the impact that environmental toxins have on cardiovascular health.

Treacherous tobacco

Smoking is probably the single most dangerous thing you can do to your body. I am well aware that nicotine is a highly addictive substance and breaking the habit is extremely difficult. Nevertheless, do whatever is necessary to stop smoking. It is urgent. It is deadly.

Tobacco smoke is the most important contributor to indoor air pollution. Whether smoked, chewed or inhaled via secondhand smoke, tobacco heightens the risk of a heart attack. People who are exposed to secondhand smoke for anywhere from one to seven hours a week increase their risk for a heart attack by 24 percent. Smoking tobacco not only increases cardiovascular risk by itself, but in combination with other risk factors risk escalates dramatically. Smoking also increases blood pressure and the tendency for blood to clot. Moreover, most people are unaware that smoking decreases HDL cholesterol.

Nicotine is partially to blame for these ill effects. It temporarily increases blood pressure, heart rate and blood flow from the heart. It can also cause arteries to narrow. Meanwhile, carbon monoxide in tobacco smoke reduces the amount of oxygen in the blood. The combination of nicotine and carbon monoxide creates an imbalance between cells' increased demand for oxygen and the reduced amount of oxygen the blood can supply.

Perilous particulates

Polluted outdoor air contains a toxic stew of fine particles and gases, as well as the ozone formed when pollutants interact with sunlight. Chemicals in these particles include the byproducts of burning gasoline, coal, wood and garbage, such as carbon monoxide, carbon dioxide, smog-forming nitrogen oxides and carcinogens like benzene and polyaromatic hydrocarbons. Add to that dust, ash, lead and other heavy metals as well as other toxins. Air pollution actually accounts for a significant number of cases of cardiovascular disease. Arsenic exposure, mostly from industrial fumes, is a potential risk factor for atherosclerosis.

The pollution levels in many American cities can trigger abnormal heart rhythms and sudden heart attacks as well as contribute to atherosclerosis, cause inflammation of heart tissue and even thicken the blood. "Environmental cardiology" is a new term coined for this new medical specialty. According to the Environmental Protection Agency (EPA), warmer temperatures resulting from global warming can also exacerbate heart disease.

It is not fully understood just how airborne pollutants damage the heart, but inflammation definitely appears to be involved. The minute particles irritate the lungs, provoking an immune system response, which in turn leads to processes that result in arterial restriction and atherosclerosis. Animal studies show that tiny particulates can trigger the formation of free radicals in the lungs and heart, which also cause inflammation. These particulates can also stimulate the production of C-reactive protein, which can cause inflammation linked to increased risk of cardiovascular disease. In addition to inflammation, particulates increase production of fibrinogen, thus thickening the blood and increasing its tendency to form clots. It also appears that particulates (and ozone) can slow heart rate, especially in individuals with hypertension, CAD and diabetes.

A recent study by American Cancer Society suggests that long-term exposure to fine particulates in the air at present levels in North America will lead to an increased cardiovascular mortality risk (primarily in the form of heart attacks and strokes) of 12 percent for every 10 micrometers of particulate matter within one cubic meter of air, resulting in an estimated 60,000 deaths a year. This number could be cut if the federal government were willing to restrict carbon dioxide emissions.

In simple terms, if you live within a mile of a major highway, you likely have high levels of particulate matter in your home. People who live near a major highway, where air is most polluted, are at increased risk for death from stroke and heart attack. There are companies that can come in and check your home for toxic exposure. You can determine outdoor particulate quality by going to the Environmental Protection Agency's website, www.epa.gov, for local air quality daily forecasts and information on indoor air quality monitors.

Heavy metals

About three years ago, a study published by the *Journal of the American Medical Association* made the headlines. It stated that men with the highest levels of mercury had a 50 percent increase in sudden cardiac death. Mercury as well as all toxic metals levels must be checked on in everyone. The detoxification chapter offers a detailed discussion of this.

Even moderate exposure to lead can cause hypertension. In fact, after genetics, exposure to lead is the most common cause of high blood pressure, more so than salt intake or aging. Lead is also implicated in heart attacks and strokes.

CHAPTER 8

Exercise Is Essential

Inactivity and excess weight tend to go together, but not exercising in and of itself can increase your risk of having cardiovascular problems. In other words, your weight can be normal but if your fitness program consists of lifting your fork and changing channels with the remote, you're putting yourself at risk. On the flip side, numerous studies have shown that half an hour to an hour of physical activity on most days reduces the risk of CAD.

Physical inactivity alone increases the risk of hypertension by 30 percent. Research has shown that following a long-term aerobic exercise program can control blood pressure as effectively as drugs do. In one study, middle-aged adults who engaged in aerobic exercise for two hours a week over an 18-month period reduced their average blood pressure and further reduced it over another 18 months, even in those who did not significantly change their weight.

In addition to helping to keep your weight under control by reducing body fat and building muscle, a regular exercise program minimizes the risk of developing or worsening existing heart disease, hypertension and high cholesterol. A fitness program also helps you maintain healthy bones, joints and muscles so you can continue to exercise and reap its benefits as you age.

When you work out may be just as important as how much. For about four hours after a fatty meal, arteries lose their ability to expand and contract in response to an increase in blood flow. A new study suggests that by exercising within two hours *after* a high-fat meal, you can reverse both the arterial dysfunction caused by the oxidation of fatty foods and actually make your arteries healthier and more flexible than they were *before* the meal.

Aerobic exercise

Any activity that raises your heart rate—running, jogging, walking fast or playing singles tennis—is particularly valuable for cardiovascular health. Aerobic activities increase your intake of oxygen, thus oxygenating your blood. Because your heart is pumping more blood each minute, with each stroke your heart is enhancing its ability to carry more oxygenated blood to muscles. Aerobic exercise can help control high blood pressure, increase "good" HDL cholesterol and reduce triglyceride levels. It also helps reduce insulin resistance, which as you will learn in a later chapter, is also important to weight control and prevention of diabetes.

Those who are not jocks will be pleased to know that brisk walking has been shown to help prevent CAD. And all of you who say you don't have time to exercise have lost your excuse: three 10-minute sessions each day have been shown to be almost as effective as one half-hour session in preventing coronary heart disease. You can do one before work, one at lunch hour and one after work with virtually no pain.

Strength training

The other component of exercise, called strength training or anaerobic exercise, includes working with weights or doing isometrics. It works synergistically with aerobic exercise to reduce body fat, increase muscle mass, reduce high blood pressure and improve cholesterol levels as well as build strength and enhance flexibility. One bonus in building muscle is that muscle tissue burns calories faster than fat does, helping with weight control.

CHAPTER 9

The Importance of Diet

A diet high in fat, particularly saturated fat, is typically blamed for the development of cardiovascular disease and salting food is often blamed for high blood pressure. Both these factors have been oversimplified.

While I am not advocating a diet dominated by fatty meats doused with salt, my dietary approach to preventing CAD, stroke and hypertension is based upon the pioneering work of Dr. Robert Atkins. Namely, you should watch your overall carbohydrate intake, eat only "good" carbs, avoid processed foods, eat a variety of protein sources and rely on organic foods as much as possible. In moderation, salt is usually not problematic because eating plenty of vegetables, as I recommend, will supply the potassium, calcium and potassium that naturally lower your blood pressure.

Excess body fat results from taking in more calories than your body needs for its metabolic activities. Dietary fat doesn't turn into body fat unless it is part of an overall pattern of over-consumption and under-utilization of fuel.

There is significant evidence that eating large amounts of refined carbohydrates that comprise much of the typical American diet can set up a cycle of blood sugar highs and lows that lead to overeating, while dietary fat actually depresses appetite because it provides the sensation of satiety. It is simple carbs that are converted to fat, not fatty foods.

The role of fat

As I mentioned before, dietary fat is often depicted as a villain, but it should not be confused with the fat on our hips and stomachs, which *is* a health hazard. We *need* fat to sustain life to build cell membranes and make hemoglobin to transport oxygen in red blood cells and produce chemicals that help regulate many of the body's functions. Fats, or fatty acids as scientists call them, can be divided into three basic types based on their chemical makeup:

* *Saturated fats*, such as butter, suet and lard, are usually solid at room temperature and are primarily animal fats, but a few, like palm and coconut oil, come from plants and are liquid at room temperature;

* *Monounsaturated fats*, found in olive oil, nuts and seeds and avocados, are liquid at room temperature;

* *Polyunsaturated fats*, also liquid at room temperature, are found in corn, canola, safflower, soybean and flaxseed oils, as well as the oil in fatty, cold-water fish.

There is general agreement that eating so-called "good" fats such as olive oil and cold-water fish promote good health. But it is simplistic to associate certain foods with one kind of fat. All natural fats, whether from animals or plants, contain a mix of fatty acids. For example, a broiled hamburger contains 39 percent saturated and 43 percent monounsaturated fat. The important thing is to eat a balance of fats. So, for example, if you're eating red meat or poultry for dinner, be sure to dress your vegetables with olive oil instead of butter and perhaps top your salad with a handful of walnuts.

The confusion over saturated fat

Eating saturated fat is said to increase the amount of cholesterol in blood, while eating polyunsaturated fat decreases it.

Monounsaturated fat doesn't raise cholesterol levels and may decrease them. Population studies of Mediterranean cultures such as the Greeks, who rely heavily on olive oil, or African cultures in which peanuts are an important component (both contain monounsaturated fats), have traditionally had extremely low rates of CAD. But the traditional diet of Aleutians (Eskimos), which relies heavily on saturated fat in the form of seal blubber, is also associated with low rates of heart disease, as is the case with the Masai tribesmen of Africa, who subsist in large part on meat, blood and fermented milk.

Saturated fat also supposedly increases the amount of triglycerides in the blood. Sugar and simple carbohydrates are the cause of elevated triglycerides, not the consumption of saturated fat. Because elevated blood levels of both LDL cholesterol and triglycerides are associated with atherosclerosis, which can lead to CAD, saturated fats have been demonized. But let's take a closer look. The studies upon which the theory that saturated fat raised cholesterol is based did not take into consideration that the subjects were also eating lots of refined carbohydrates. A diet high in *both* saturated fat and low-quality carbohydrates is definitely associated with high blood cholesterol. But until recently, no research looked at the impact of saturated fat without a heavy carbohydrate load. Nor did most of the original studies on saturated fat take organic fats and fats from grass-fed meats into consideration or the fact that some people who eat a lot of meat don't eat many vegetables and fruits. So tobacco smoke or the absence of the phytonutrients in produce, rather than the presence of saturated fat, may have been responsible for the high cholesterol levels and increased risk for heart disease.

Some studies show that even when carbohydrates are not limited, although a moderate amount of saturated fat raises LDL ("bad") cholesterol levels, its effect is cancelled out by a comparable rise in the level of HDL ("good") cholesterol. It also appears that eating a high-fat diet, including saturated fat, has little or no impact on the risk of stroke.

Low-carb vs. low-fat

A recent spate of studies that compared high-fat diets with low-fat diets have confirmed the life's work of Dr. Atkins, who championed a low-carbohydrate dietary approach and advised only the avoidance of trans fats found in hydrogenated and partially hydrogenated oils.

In one clinical trial, researchers compared triglyceride and other blood cholesterol levels of 19 normal weight men who already had high triglycerides after putting them first on a high-fat/low-carbohydrate diet and then a low-fat/high-carbohydrate one. After following the high-fat diet for three weeks, the men had decreased their triglyceride levels by an average of 63 percent, their total cholesterol by 22 percent. After three weeks on the low-fat diet, the good results were generally reversed. The men had increased their triglyceride levels by an average of 63 percent and their VLDL levels by 19 percent. For people who already have high triglycerides, cutting down on fat and relying heavily on carbohydrates only makes a bad situation worse. The counterintuitive higher-fat diet is clearly preferable.

A number of other studies have found comparable results that strengthen the argument that it is not fat but excessive carbohydrates that raise LDL cholesterol and triglycerides, which can lead to atherosclerosis and CAD. Additionally, more people seem able to stick with low-carb diet programs than the low-fat ones.

Essential fatty acids

Essential fatty acids are fats that your body needs but cannot manufacture itself and must get from food or dietary supplements. Found in polyunsaturated fats, they include omega-3 fatty acids (or alpha linolenic acids) and omega-6 fatty acids (or gamma linoleic acids). It is not just eating these fats that is important, it is also crucial that we have a balance of the two.

The typical American diet, which is full of cheap vegetable oils, tends to give us more than enough omega-6s, while leaving us deficient in the omega-3s found in cold-water fish and flaxseed oil, as well as in fish oil and blue green algae supplements. Both types can reduce levels of dangerous blood lipids, but omega-3s are the ones that can thin the blood and reduce the likelihood of a stroke or heart attack.

Trans fats are bad fats

There is one form of fat that is unequivocally dangerous. Unlike other fats, trans fats are manufactured, chemically altered fats. Eating them in the form of hydrogenated or partially hydrogenated oils found in most margarines, peanut butter, baked goods and fried foods and many other processed foods hits your body with a triple whammy: it elevates LDL and triglyceride levels and reduces HDL levels. But the damage from these artificial fats doesn't stop there. Research shows that they also increase the number of small, dense, sticky Type B LDL particles, and the higher the trans fat content of the diet, the smaller the particles and the higher your risk of CAD.

In this same study, subjects also ate a comparison diet in which the fat came from butter, a saturated fat without any trans fats. Interestingly, although butter produced the highest cholesterol levels, it also provided the highest proportion of "good" large, fluffy LDL particles.

Trans fats also make blood vessels less flexible, increasing the susceptibility to atherosclerosis. But major studies have shown that even a small amount of trans fats in the diet can increase the risk of CAD. These and other studies led to the Food and Drug Administration (FDA) finally mandating that food manufacturers list amounts of trans fats on food labels, effective in 2006.

Remember, no amount of trans fat is safe. You can avoid them by reading nutritional labels and looking for their pseudonyms: hydrogenated and partially hydrogenated oil.

Cities across the country have responded to the danger of trans fats by banning them from restaurant kitchens. Responsible manufacturers are also making a good faith effort to remove trans fats (a.k.a. shortening or margarine) from prepared foods including baked goods.

The role of carbohydrates

Eating carbohydrates quickly raises blood sugar (glucose), which in turn prompts the release of insulin to transport the glucose not immediately needed for energy to the cells. If there is more glucose than you need, the remainder is stored in the liver and muscles as glycogen.

> *It's not fat that causes you to get fat, it's sugar and simple carbs.*

Once these storage areas are full, any additional glucose is stored as fat. This body fat comes from excess carbohydrates, as well as excess protein and dietary fat. In other words, it's not fat that causes you to get fat, it's sugar and simple carbs.

All these processes are perfectly normal and allowed our ancestors to store fat so they could survive in times of famine. But most of us feast daily and have never experienced a famine, so the fat accumulates, creating a major risk factor for CAD, stroke and hypertension. Blood sugar and insulin play another important role in the development of these conditions and of diabetes.

The seesaw of blood sugar and insulin

When you regularly overeat and much of your diet is made up of carbohydrates, blood sugar levels constantly challenge your pancreas to produce insulin. Over time, this mechanism can become stressed, requiring more and more insulin. Eventually, the insulin may be ineffective, leading to a condition called insulin resistance that lays the groundwork for pre-diabetes and ultimately Type 2 diabetes.

People with insulin resistance, pre-diabetes or diabetes are also at increased risk of developing heart disease and stroke. The risks are even greater when they are also associated with obesity—particularly belly fat—hypertension, abnormal cholesterol and high triglycerides. Even before the onset of diabetes, resistance to insulin is linked to atherosclerosis. Study after study links high insulin levels with increased risk for heart attacks. Most people with high blood pressure also have high triglyceride and high insulin levels.

There is no better way to control blood sugar and insulin levels than to moderate your carbohydrate intake and focus on nutrient-rich, unrefined carbohydrates, primarily in the form of vegetables. By eating this way, you can also reduce "bad" (LDL) cholesterol, raise "good" (HDL) cholesterol and reduce triglycerides, all without being obsessive about fat (other than trans fats).

Heart-friendly foods

Most vegetables and some fruits are low in carbohydrates and rank low in the glycemic index. They're full of fiber, antioxidants, vitamins and minerals, all of which benefit your cardiovascular system. A population study of almost 10,000 Americans who had been tracked for almost two decades found that those who ate vegetables and fruits three or more times a day had a 42 percent lower risk of dying from a stroke, a 27 percent lower risk of dying from cardiovascular disease and a 24 percent lower risk of dying from CAD than those who ate produce only once a day or not at all.

In addition to the general run of fresh vegetables and fruits, the following foods are particularly effective at reducing cholesterol and providing nutrients that protect your arteries:

- **Yogurt** contains probiotics that reduce bile acids, which helps keep cholesterol from being absorbed from the gastrointestinal tract. Be sure to eat only yogurt with active lactobacillus cultures and without any added sugar or sweetened fruit.

- **Salmon** is rich in omega-3 fatty acids that thin the blood, reducing the risk of heart attack or stroke. They also decrease triglyceride levels, lower blood pressure, inhibit the growth of plaque, and protect against irregular heartbeat, which can cause heart attacks. Be sure to choose wild salmon rather than the farm-raised type, which is not as high in omega-3s and contains antibiotics and other toxins.

- **Spinach**, kale, and other dark leafy vegetables help prevent cardiovascular disease in several ways. They are superb sources of the antioxidant vitamins C and A, the latter in the form of beta-carotene. The former is water soluble and the latter fat soluble; as a team, they help prevent the oxidization of cholesterol, which contributes to atherosclerosis and can result in a heart attack or stroke. Spinach is also an excellent source of folate, which neutralizes homocysteine. High levels of homocysteine are an independent risk factor for a heart attack or stroke. Spinach is also rich in magnesium, as well as certain peptides, all of which help lower high blood pressure. Magnesium also protects against heart disease.

- **Almonds** are full of vitamin E and omega-3 fatty acids, which have been shown to help prevent CAD, stroke and hypertension, by helping to thin the blood. Most of the fat in almonds is the monounsaturated variety that helps lower LDL cholesterol.

- **Garlic** can slow the development of atherosclerosis.

The benefits of alcohol—in moderation

The old saw about moderation in all things could not be truer in the case of alcohol.

Regular heavy consumption, meaning three or more drinks a day, puts you at risk for hemorrhagic stroke and hypertension and can damage the heart muscle. Occasional binge drinking can cause accelerated heartbeat (atrial fibrillation) that could trigger a heart attack or stroke in a person with underlying heart disease. Individuals who have had a heart attack can further damage their heart and develop high blood pressure even with moderate drinking.

On the other hand, abstainers actually have roughly twice the chance of having a stroke than do moderate drinkers. For some, moderate alcohol use seems to offer protection against cardiovascular disease. By moderate, we are talking about no more than one drink a day for women or two for men. One drink is equivalent to a bottle or can of beer or wine cooler, 5 ounces of wine or 1.5 ounces of liquor. Moderate use can also lower blood pressure. Overall, moderate drinkers are less likely to have a heart attack than heavy drinkers or non-drinkers. Moderate alcohol consumption has equal opportunity benefits, regardless of age, race or sex.

The specific benefits of moderate consumption include:

- Elevating levels of HDL cholesterol

- Decreasing levels of LDL cholesterol

- Reducing triglycerides

- Reducing blood pressure

- Providing antioxidant effects, by countering the oxidation of LDL cholesterol, which damages arteries

- Inhibiting the formation of blood clots that can lead to stroke or heart attack

- Helping prevent arterial constriction, increasing coronary blood flow

- Reducing levels of insulin in the blood

- Reducing inflammation

Wine, spirits or beer?

Most of the heart protective effects of alcohol are due to the ethanol in all alcoholic beverages but increasingly researchers are looking at the effects of other components. Like wine, moderate intake of beer lowers LDL cholesterol and triglycerides and reduces the tendency for blood to clot, but whether its benefits match those of wine are in dispute. A study of more than 13,000 Danish men and women indicates that those who drink wine have a lower risk of stroke than those who don't, but no similar connection exists between reduced risk and drinking either beer or spirits. Drinking wine apparently helps reduce levels of fibrinogen in the blood.

Until recently, the assumption was that the antioxidant benefit in wine came primarily from the antioxidants in grape skins, with the result that red wine was considered more heart protective. However, laboratory tests now suggest that those who prefer white wine can also get a similar boost because the pulp is just as rich in other antioxidants.

How about coffee?

Coffee is also full of antioxidants, but go easy on the caffeine, particularly if you are not a regular coffee hound. A cup of java can give you a bigger jolt than you bargained for, according to a recent Costa Rican study of individuals who had suffered nonfatal heart attacks. The study suggests that people who normally drink no more than a cup a day have a four-fold increase in their chances of having a heart attack within an hour after drinking coffee.

Coffee also seems to pose more of risk for people with other risk factors for heart disease, such as being inactive or smoking. In fact, those with three or more risk factors more than doubled their risk after a cup of coffee. Caffeine apparently causes a brief surge in blood pressure and heightened activity in the nervous system that could trigger a heart attack.

People who drink lots of coffee have a greater risk of a certain kind of stroke, known as an aneurysmal subarachnoid hemorrhage (SAH). A Norwegian population study of more than 27,000 people showed that those who drank more than five cups were almost two and a half times more likely to suffer an SAH.

CHAPTER 10

The Salerno Solution Heart Disease Supplement Program

Although I will discuss several individual nutrients, it is important to remember that supplements work best as part of an overall program. This point is brought home in a five-year study conducted in the Chinese province of Linxian that examined the impact of supplements on people 60 years and older who had high systolic blood pressure, putting them at elevated risk for stroke. Individuals who took supplements containing vitamin A, zinc, beta-carotene, selenium and the alpha-tocopherol form of vitamin E had a reduction in their risk of stroke of 29 percent compared to controls that did not take them.

Omega-3 fatty acids

I recommend fish oil for everyone, and it is especially important for people with heart disease.

There is overwhelming evidence that omega-3 fatty acids, particularly fish oils, have been consistently shown to reduce the risk of strokes and fatal and non-fatal heart attacks in a number of ways. Fish oils help keep artery walls flexible, reduce the process of plaque growth, reduce triglyceride levels, prevent blood clotting, reduce blood pressure and stabilize heart rhythm.

Fish oil appears to help prevent arrhythmia and sudden heart attack in healthy men as well as cut the risk of another heart attack, stroke or death for individuals who have already had a heart attack. Many studies have confirmed that fish oil can also lower blood pressure in people with hypertension.

A recent study of the benefits of omega-3 fatty acids reviewed 48 earlier studies and concluded that consuming cold-water fish or taking fish oil supplements significantly reduced the risk for heart attack, stroke and sudden death, as well as overall mortality.

People who eat fatty, cold-water fish also appear to have lower levels of C-reactive protein (CRP), high levels of which signal inflammation and contribute to plaque in blood vessels. A recent Japanese study found that the more cold-water fish that elderly men and women ate, the lower their blood levels of CRP.

If you are a vegetarian, you can get omega-3s from flaxseed and flaxseed oil, but the absorption is somewhat lower, so you may need to take more.

Optimal daily dose: 1,000–2,000 mg. *Note:* Must be mercury-free guaranteed by the producer. If you are on blood thinners like Coumadin, consult your doctor before starting fish oil. It can further thin your blood to dangerous levels, so your dosage may need to be adjusted.

Coenzyme Q-10 (Co Q-10)

This essential nutrient is also recommended for everyone and it also plays a special role for people with heart disease.

Extreme deficiency of Co Q-10 can lead to impaired energy production, oxidative stress and cardiac failure. Not only do the body's stores of Co Q-10 become depleted with age, people with heart disease are often deficient in it. Statin drugs that many people are prescribed to control their cholesterol actually deplete stores of Co Q-10, so supplementation is essential if you are taking statin drugs like Lipitor or Crestor.

Moreover, people with elevated cholesterol levels tend to have lower levels of Co Q-10 than healthy people of the same age.

The endothelium is the layer of cells on the inner surface of blood vessels. When all is well in endothelial vascular cells, they dilate and constrict easily in response to the heart's beats. A healthy endothelium also makes the formation of clots less likely. But atherosclerosis, elevated cholesterol, CAD and diabetes all wreak havoc with vascular endothelial function. Research on diabetic patients with abnormal lipid levels experienced improved vascular dilation after 12 weeks of daily supplementation with 200 mgs a day of Co Q-10.

More than a third of people with hypertension are deficient in Co Q-10. Happily, the antioxidant lowers blood pressure in patients with hypertension.

Optimal daily dose: 100–200 mg. *Note:* Consult your doctor if you are taking blood thinners, because, like fish oil, Co Q-10 can thin your blood to dangerous levels if you take too much in combination with pharmaceuticals like Coumadin.

Vitamin E

A fat-soluble antioxidant, vitamin E is believed to help prevent diseases associated with oxidative stress, including cardiovascular disease.

It now appears that doses of vitamin E ranging from more than 300 mgs to as much as 1,000 mgs a day may help prevent the plaque buildup that leads to atherosclerosis. It seems clearer that vitamin E is effective in reducing high blood pressure.

Optimal daily dose: 400–1,000 units. Look for a mixed tocopherol and tocotrienol form to be assured of optimal antioxidant performance plus tocotrienols help in lowering triglycerides, reducing plaque and improving cellular health.

Vitamin C

Vitamin C is valuable in general and particularly for cardiovascular health in large part because of its antioxidant properties. It is also necessary for building collagen and the integrity of your body's tissues, including your arteries.

Dr. Linus Pauling regarded atherosclerosis as a disease caused by the deficiency of vitamin C. If your intake of vitamin C is inadequate, the blood vessels in the endothelium weaken; in response, lipoprotein(a) forms and bonds to the arterial walls in an effort to strengthen them. Lipoprotein(a) increases the amount of "bad" cholesterol in your arteries, exacerbating the development of plaque. However, among its many benefits, treatment with vitamin C has been shown to reverse blood vessel dysfunction.

Extensive research on vitamin C has confirmed its cardio-protective benefits. A recent study pooled analyses from nine studies, comprising 290,000 individuals who did not initially have CAD and who were followed for an average of 10 years. Results showed that subjects who consumed more than 700 mgs a day of supplemental vitamin C had a 25 percent lower risk of CHD than those who did not take vitamin C supplements.

The lower the blood levels of vitamin C, the greater also the risk of suffering a stroke, according to a 20-year study of more than 2,100 Japanese men and women. Those who ate vegetables six or seven days a week had a 54 percent lower risk of stroke than those who ate them no more than two days a week or not at all. Risk of death from stroke in older people is also inversely associated with blood levels of vitamin C, according to a 20-year study in Great Britain.

Vitamin C is also effective in lowering blood pressure in people with moderate hypertension. Taking 500 mgs of vitamin C daily for a month lowered blood pressure by up to 9.1 percent.

It's a good idea to include high C-content fruits and vegetables in your daily diet as well.

Optimal daily dose: 500–3,000 mg of a product that contains Ester-C, which is more absorbable and less acidic.

Garlic extract

Both allicin and the organosulfur compounds in garlic benefit the cardiovascular system in a number of ways. Garlic helps manage cholesterol by decreasing its synthesis in the liver. Finally, it appears that organosulfur compounds can stimulate the synthesis of the antioxidant glutathione. Many studies have shown that garlic can help prevent or control mild hypertension.

Optimal daily dose: 200 mg of an aged garlic extract. *Note:* Garlic can thin the blood so it should not be combined with prescription blood-thinners such as Coumadin.

Nattokinase

Nattokinase is an enzyme extracted from natto, a traditional Japanese food made from fermented soybeans. The properties of nattokinase closely resemble those of plasmin, a clot dissolving enzyme your body produces. This means that nattokinase dissolves fibrin, which encourages clotting directly. It also enhances the effects of plasmin and other clot-dissolving agents. Nattokinase both thins the blood so clots are less likely to develop and helps dissolves existing clots, which can cause heart attacks and stroke.

There have been numerous animal studies and several on humans, all demonstrating the effectiveness of nattokinase in dissolving clots.

A blend of nattokinase and pychnogenol has been shown to reduce the likelihood of deep vein thrombosis (potentially fatal blood clots) on long airplane flights.

Optimal daily dose: Up to 100 mg. *Note:* Like fish oil and Co Q-10, nattokinase can thin blood to dangerous levels if you are taking blood thinners.

I'm adding the following list of supplements that have been scientifically validated to have important heart protective benefits. Please discuss them with your health care practitioner.

In addition to the basic supplements mentioned in Section 1, here are some supplements you should discuss with your health care provider to determine which ones are right for you and your condition. Many of these are described in detail in this book.

- Bromelain

- Carnitine

- Resveratrol/red wine extract

- Green tea extract

- Magnesium

- Vitamin B complex that includes:

  - Vitamin B_6: 20 mg

  - Vitamin B_{12}: 1 mg

  - Vitamin B_3: Niacin (slow release): 500 mg

- Folic acid: 800 mcg

- Selenium

- N-acetylcholine

- Chlorella

- Grapeseed extract

CHAPTER 11

Protect and Prevent

The following strategies will help reduce your risks for CAD, stroke and hypertension:

- Lose weight if you are overweight (a BMI of more than 24.9).

- Exercise for a minimum of half an hour most days of the week.

- Don't smoke or expose yourself to secondhand smoke.

- Don't drink alcohol in excess. (one drink for women and two for men daily is OK).

- Obtain most of your carbohydrates from fresh, organic vegetables and some fruit. Eat at least four cups of vegetables daily.

- Supplement your diet with cardio-protective nutrients.

- Don't eat foods made with trans fats. Read labels. Watch out for shortening, margarine, hydrogenated oils and other euphemisms for trans fats.

- Know your blood pressure and check it routinely.

- Have your cholesterol levels checked on a regular basis and ask your health care provider about also monitoring your pattern B LDL, triglycerides, homocysteine, and other markers.

- Practice good dental hygiene and see your dentist at least twice a year for regular checkups.

- To avoid environmental toxins, don't run or engage in other exercise beside major highways.

- Make sure fireplaces and wood burning and gas stoves are well ventilated.

THE TOP EIGHT CHANGES YOU CAN MAKE TODAY TO PREVENT HEART DISEASE, STROKE, AND HYPERTENSION

Let's cut right to the chase: **Heart disease, hypertension and stroke are nearly 95 percent preventable.** Be sure to read all the detailed information in this chapter to access complete information on each change listed below.

1. **Cut out white flour, refined carbohydrates of any kind and sugars and artificial sweeteners of any kind** and you are well on your way to better heart function.

   Refined carbs and sugar raises insulin levels, which cause waxy deposits in the coronary arteries, carotid arteries and kidneys. They also increase the likelihood that your blood will clot.

2. **Avoid trans fats.** Be wary of hidden trans fats in bakery goods and prepared foods. This is a particularly deadly form of fat that will clog arteries and increase blood viscosity.

3. **Ensure that your homocysteine level is below 8 mm/L.** Homocysteine is a protein in our blood which, when elevated, will increase the likelihood of clogged arteries. We should all take vitamin B_6 (20 mg), B_{12} (1 mg), and folic acid (800 mcg) to ensure homocysteine is low.

4. **Eat four to six servings (cups) of organic fruits and vegetables of the non-starchy kind every single day.** Berries are the best fruits as are nonstarchy vegetables like broccoli, spinach, kale, tomatoes and peppers.

5. **Eat three servings of low mercury fish a week.** Wild caught (never farmed!) salmon, mahi mahi, halibut and most shellfish are the best low mercury choices. Also take 2,000 mg in fish oil supplements a day. If you are taking aspirin or blood thinner, see a doctor. You must reduce your dose.

6. **Maintain triglyceride levels below 100.** A low-carb diet, fish oil and slow-release niacin (around 500 mg) per day are recommended. Getting your HDL levels above 50 through diet and exercise (20–30 minutes per day for five days a week) are also desirable.

7. **Moderate strength training two to four days per week is also beneficial.** Ten minutes of lifting five-pound weights is a good start. You can find an excellent video that teaches you basic strength training exercises and techniques at Michele Smith's website: www.foreverfitwithmichele.com.

8. **Have your mercury, lead, and cadmium levels checked.** The *Journal of the American Medical Association* showed that men with the highest level of mercury had a 50 percent increased risk of dying from heart disease. Lead and cadmium can elevate blood pressure and have other serious consequences. Selenium (200 mcg per day) and N-acetyl cysteine (600 mg per day) as well as chlorella (200 mg per day) are good oral chelating agents and will insure that these heavy metals will not accumulate. Intravenous chelation also protects from heart disease.

Preventing and Treating Type 2 Diabetes

Mrs. T came to my center suffering from moderate obesity and Type 2 diabetes. She was taking nearly 100 units of insulin and was on Glucophage, a drug used to lower glucose levels. She was having difficulty losing weight, her blood sugars still averaged around 170, and she was tired all the time and depressed. She was only 48 years old.

When she first came to the Salerno Center, extensive blood tests were taken including insulin and glucose levels fasting and two hours after eating a high carb meal. Mrs. T's insulin levels were through the roof as were her glucose levels. Her thyroid gland was underactive, she had a huge amount of candida fungus in her blood and her triglycerides were extremely elevated. Neither is typical for people with diabetes. More typically, her blood pressure was also high. This poor women was a stroke or heart attack waiting to happen.

I placed Mrs. T immediately on a low-carb, yeast-free diet where most cheeses, vinegar and mushrooms were eliminated along with virtually all sugars. She was placed on Salerno Multi-Vitamin, Anti-Aging Factor and probiotic for yeast as well as Salerno Blood Pressure Factor to lower her elevated blood pressure. She was also given fish oil to lower her triglyceride level. High triglycerides are a bigger risk factor for stroke and heart disease (especially in women) than cholesterol levels. The fish oil was also given to help thin her too-thick blood that additionally increased her risk of a stroke or heart attack.

She was also placed on a thyroid medication. Her insulin injections were reduced to accommodate her new diet and vitamin regimen. After just a week, Mrs. T lost four pounds, and her insulin requirement decreased another 15 percent. Mrs. T was feeling more energetic and less depressed. She lost another four pounds the following week and continued to reduce her insulin to about one-fourth of her starting level. By week 16, Mrs. T was completely off her insulin and had lost 36 pounds. She said she felt "great," better than she had felt in years and she was beginning a running program. Mrs. T's triglycerides had normalized, her blood pressure was perfect and by week 48, she was even off her Glucophage medication.

Cases like these number in the hundreds at the Salerno Center. A modified version of the diet and supplementation program could cut the risk of Type 2 diabetes by over 95 percent in the general population and even reverse it in many cases.

CHAPTER 12

What Is Diabetes?

At its most simple, diabetes is a disorder of the glucose metabolism. In plain English, this means that you have diabetes when your body is unable to quickly and efficiently balance the blood sugar produced by the body's natural process of digesting sugar and other carbohydrates.

Consider the classic American dinner of macaroni and cheese casserole with a side salad. The noodles, cheese, milk-based sauce and breadcrumbs are chock full of carbohydrates along with fat and protein. The salad vegetables contain more carbohydrates (although these are the good carbs). Commercially prepared salad dressings often contain more carbohydrates and fat.

The starchy carbohydrates in the noodles and bread crumbs begin to break down into glucose almost the moment you put them in your mouth. Salad vegetables take longer to break down. The entire process of digesting carbs is completed in your digestive system. (Protein and fat break down more slowly.) Your body functions within a fairly narrow blood sugar level range, so as highly processed carbohydrate foods begin to convert to glucose and your blood sugar level rises, your pancreas releases the hormone insulin.

The job of insulin is to ferry blood sugar from your blood stream to your cells, where it can be converted to energy. Any extra blood sugar is converted to glycogen and stored in the liver and muscle cells for use at a later date. *When the glycogen storage areas are full, the remaining glucose is stored as body fat.* With fuel for immediate energy needs, plus two auxiliary storage areas—glycogen for the short term and body fat for the long term—this backup system allowed early man to survive for reasonably long periods when food was in short supply.

Feast or famine

Obviously, things have changed over the millennia. For most of us, the closest you ever get to a period of famine is the 12 or so hours between dinner and breakfast. Nor do you expend vast amounts of energy traveling everywhere on foot tracking game and trying to keep warm without central heating. So if you continue to eat like a caveman without the caveman's lifestyle, you're going to plump up. Too many carbs will tax your pancreas and that can lead to Type 2 diabetes.

The differences between Type 1 and Type 2 diabetes

Diabetes mellitus, both Types 1 and 2, are diseases that prevent your body from properly using the energy from the food you eat. Type 1 diabetes occurs when the pancreas (an organ behind your stomach) produces little insulin or no insulin at all. It is usually discovered in childhood and requires insulin for the sufferer's survival.

Type 2 diabetes can be thought of as a lifestyle disease which occurs when the pancreas makes insulin, but the insulin does not work to balance blood sugar as it should because an improper diet and lack of exercise creates insulin resistance.

Often, I find my patients confuse Types 1 and 2 diabetes. Type 1 diabetes, also known as juvenile diabetes, can develop at any age, however it most commonly appears in children, adolescents and young adults and is a result of a malfunctioning pancreas.

Type 2, once called adult-onset diabetes, results from a pancreas that has been exhausted by a bad diet and lack of exercise. Almost all people with Type 2 diabetes are overweight or obese.

Type 2 diabetes is one of the most alarming epidemics in our country today. It now reaches into the childhood population to inflict its deadly consequences. This is one malady that can be linked inextricably to our Western diet and life of inactivity. On the flip side, it is one ailment that is almost completely preventable, provided you take a proactive stance against it.

Protect and prevent

The following strategies will help reduce your risks for Type 2 diabetes:

- Know whether you have a family history of the disease.

- Lose weight if you are overweight (a BMI of more than 24.9). Exercise for a minimum of half an hour most days of the week.

- Don't drink alcohol in excess or at all if you have problems with unbalanced blood sugar.

- Obtain most of your carbohydrates from fresh, organic vegetables and small amounts of fruit and whole grains.

- Supplement your diet with recommended nutrients.

- After age 45, have your blood sugar levels checked every three years or more frequently if you are at risk. Overweight children should be under the close supervision of a medical professional to monitor blood glucose levels. Ballooning rates of Type 2 diabetes have become an indictment of our lives of inactivity and over-consumption as well as our reliance on sweets, soft drinks and other junk foods full of empty carbohydrates. The U.S. is ranked third in the number of cases of Type 2 diabetes in the world and number one among Western/

industrialized nation. Here are some 2012 facts from the International Diabetes Federation:

- Diabetes affects more than 371 million people worldwide. This number is increasing in every country and by 2030 is expected to affect 552 million globally.

- The greatest number of people with diabetes is between 40 and 59 years of age.

- 78,000 children develop Type 1 diabetes every year.

- By 2030 estimates show that globally there will be 275 million women with diabetes.

The International Diabetes Federation has data for 216 countries and territories grouped into seven regions and reports for 2012 include these distressing statistics:

- More than 38.4 million people (11 percent of adults) in the North America region have diabetes; by 2030 this is expected to rise to 51.2 million. In the U.S. alone there were 24.1 million cases in 2012.

- More than 55 million people (8.4 percent of adults) in the Europe region have diabetes; by 2030 this is expected to rise to 64 million. Europe has the highest number of children with Type 1 diabetes. Russia leads the region with 12.7 million cases of diabetes, double any other countries in this region.

- More than 132.2 million people (8 percent of adults) in the Western Pacific region have diabetes; by 2030 this is predicted to rise to 187.9 million. More people with diabetes live in this region than any other. China holds the dubious lead with 92.3 million (more than 12 times that of any other country in this region).

- More than 70.3 million people (8.7 percent of adults) in the South-East Asia region have diabetes; by 2030 this is expected to rise to 120.9 million. One-fifth of all adults living with diabetes live in this region. India leads with 63 million (more than 11 times that of any other country in this region).

- More than 14 million people (4.3 percent of adults) in the Africa region have diabetes; by 2030 this is predicted to rise to 28 million. This region has the highest percentage of people with undiagnosed diabetes (81 percent). Nigeria (3.2 million) and South Africa (2.0 million) lead in this tragic race against healthy lifestyles.

- More than 34.2 million people in the Middle East and North Africa region have diabetes; by 2030 this is expected to rise to 59.7 million. Egypt is at the top of the list with 7.5 million, but Pakistan (6.6 million) and Iran (4.5 million) follow closely.

- In 2011 4.3 million people ages 20–79 died from diabetes, accounting for 8.2 percent of mortality globally, a 13.3 percent increase over 2010.

- Every seven seconds a person dies from diabetes.

- 48 percent of deaths due to diabetes occur with people under the age of 60.

- People with diabetes have an increased risk of developing a number of serious health problems. Consistently high blood glucose levels can lead to serious diseases affecting the heart and blood vessels, eyes, kidneys and nerves. In addition, people with diabetes also have a higher risk of developing infections. In almost all high-income countries, diabetes is a leading cause of:
  1. cardiovascular disease
  2. blindness
  3. kidney failure
  4. lower limb amputation

- Diabetes is the fourth leading cause of death by disease globally.

- At least 50 percent of all people with diabetes are unaware of their condition. In some countries this figure may reach 80 percent.

- In addition to diabetes, the condition of impaired glucose tolerance (IGT), in which the blood glucose level is higher than normal but not as high as in diabetes, is also a major public health problem. People with IGT have a higher risk of developing diabetes as well as an increased risk of cardiovascular disease.

People with diabetes are two to four times more likely to develop cardiovascular disease (CVD) than people without diabetes. CVD is the number one cause of death in industrialized countries. It is also set to overtake infectious diseases as the most common cause of death in many parts of the developing world. For each risk factor present, the risk of cardiovascular death is about three times greater in people with diabetes as compared to people without the condition. Current medical treatment for Type 2 diabetes presume the person already has CVD, indicating doctors think the development of heart disease is virtually inevitable among Type 2 diabetics.

Experts predict that one-third of American children who were born in the year 2000 will develop Type 2 diabetes. Even developing countries are seeing the incidence of diabetes skyrocket. China and India are now vying for the dubious distinction of having the largest number of people with diabetes in the world, as economic growth and newfound prosperity has led to the adoption of Western eating habits and reduction in physical labor. In both societies, where malnutrition was long rampant, being plump and idle were traditionally seen as status symbols. Today in both countries obesity is fast becoming a public health issue among affluent and even middle class segments of the population. The association of diabetes with affluence in such countries is in stark contrast with the U.S., where diabetes is more common among the poor, many of whom live in urban "food deserts" where healthy food is literally unattainable.

The sequence of events that leads to diabetes

STEP 1: *Insulin Resistance*

The typical diet in the U.S. and increasingly in other industrialized countries consists of an excessive number of calories, often in the form of processed food—meaning primarily refined carbohydrates, which quickly convert to glucose. As long as you continue to eat this way, your body gets so much sugar and simple carbohydrates that it never needs to burn its fat for energy.

A rapidly expanding waistline is the first sign that diabetes may be in your future. Most people see extra pounds as a cosmetic issue, but belly fat can also gradually make you insulin resistant. That means that your cells are less responsive to the effects of insulin. It is important to state that not everyone with insulin resistance is overweight; nor does everyone who is overweight become insulin resistant, but the two are often associated. Medical science doesn't yet entirely understand why insulin resistance develops, particularly in response to excess belly fat, but inflammation appears to play a role.

STEP 2: *Insulin Resistance with Hyperinsulinism*

Because insulin becomes less effective in making the cells absorb glucose and thereby normalizing the blood sugar level, the pancreas releases more of it, resulting in elevated levels of insulin in the bloodstream.

Instead of the normal rise and fall of both blood sugar and blood insulin levels that occur after a meal, the balance has been disturbed and blood sugars remain elevated, creating a host of risks of side effects.

Now you have both insulin resistance and hyperinsulinemia meaning that after each high-carbohydrate meal, glucose levels rise, prompting a large spike in insulin, escalating that roller coaster ride of dramatically rising and falling blood sugars.

STEP 3: Insulin Resistance, Hyperinsulinism and Low Blood Sugar

As time passes, the mechanism linking insulin and blood sugar becomes increasingly inefficient. It takes longer for the pancreas to produce insulin after a meal and then it overproduces, causing the blood sugar level to drop dramatically after a heavy dose of insulin finally kicks in. The result, called reactive hypoglycemia or low blood sugar, can set off a number of symptoms such as peaks and valleys in energy, jitters, irritability and even brain fog. Cravings for sweets and other carbohydrate foods are also common as the body tries to raise its blood sugar.

STEP 4: Prediabetes

Step 3 can go on for years, but eventually the delay in insulin response causes blood sugar levels to begin to peak above the normal range. The roller coaster ride now becomes even wilder. Two hours or so after a high carb meal, the blood sugar level is higher than it should be, often provoking sleepiness. Then the insulin level spikes, resulting in the symptoms of low blood sugar described above. This trio of conditions—insulin resistance, hyperinsulinism and impaired glucose tolerance—is considered prediabetes. In my mind, it's like being "a little pregnant." Either you are or you aren't. At this point, you have diabetes. But you can change it.

STEP 5: Type 2 Diabetes with Insulin Resistance and High Insulin Production

Eventually, although the pancreas continues to overproduce insulin, it no longer works in a timely fashion, resulting in dangerously high blood sugar levels after meals.

STEP 6: *Type 2 Diabetes with Little or No Insulin* Production

Eventually, unless intervention occurs, the pancreas can no longer churn out insulin or it produces inadequate amounts. In addition to elevated after-meal blood sugar levels, fasting blood sugar levels (at least eight hours after a meal) are also in the danger zone.

According to the American Diabetes Association, a diagnosis of diabetes includes:

- a fasting blood sugar of 126 mg/dL or higher on two readings and

- a reading of 200 mg/dL or higher after a high carbohydrate meal on two occasions.

It is not until this point that many people find out that they have diabetes, often as a result of a host of symptoms that can include increases in thirst, hunger and the need to urinate. Unexplained weight gain or weight loss and blurred vision are other symptoms. Sadly, the American Diabetes Association estimates that about 30 percent of Americans with diabetes have not been diagnosed.

A worldwide epidemic

The process that leads to Type 2 diabetes can take years, but it does not necessarily proceed slowly. When you consider how most people eat and the fact that two-thirds of American adults are overweight or obese, it could seem that most of the population is likely to develop diabetes.

Although the situation is dire, this is not totally a foregone conclusion. Some people have a built-in predisposition to blood sugar and insulin imbalances while others do not. If you have such a tendency but never trigger it with overeating and eating the wrong kind of food, you may never know you have such an inclination.

That said, there is no question that diabetes has reached epidemic proportions. Just how bad is it?

- In the U.S., almost 21 million people including children—or 7 percent of the population—have diabetes, although almost one-third of them are unaware that they have the disease.

- Another 41 million have prediabetes.

- Most children who have diabetes have Type 1, which is the result of a lack of insulin caused by the destruction of beta cells in the pancreas.

- Increasingly more children have Type 2 diabetes for the same reasons adults have the disease: poor diet and lack of exercise.

This chapter focuses on Type 2 diabetes, which is preventable and, to a certain extent, reversible with lifestyle changes.

As shown in earlier statistics, the U.S. is hardly alone in its diabetes epidemic. Type 2 diabetes is on the increase globally. This trend is the most obvious in countries where social and economic changes are occurring, including the Republic of Korea, where the prevalence of diabetes increased seven-fold in 40 years, to its 2011 level of 9.9 percent. Diabetes rates in New Zealand and the Pacific Islands have doubled in the last ten years. About 7.5 percent of New Zealanders have diabetes, as do as many as 10 percent of Maoris. Residents of Hong Kong, Japan and Singapore also have especially high rates.

Diabetes is a devastating disease on its own. Diabetes is also intimately linked to a number of other serious and life-threatening conditions, including heart disease, stroke, high blood pressure, kidney disease, blindness, amputations of digits or limbs, diseases of the nervous system, gum disease, sexual dysfunction and complications of pregnancy.

Assessing your risks

A family history of diabetes is a clear message that you face an increased risk for the disease, along with several other matters beyond your control, but many critical factors are in your hands.

Age, gender and race

Although Type 2 diabetes increasingly strikes children and young adults, it is far more common in older people, particularly after age 45. Almost 21 percent of Americans aged 60 and older have diabetes. Men are slightly more likely than women to get the disease, although African American, Hispanic, Native American, Asian American and Pacific Islander women are at least two to four times more likely than non-Hispanic white women to develop it.

African Americans who do not have a Hispanic background are 1.8 times more likely to have diabetes than non-Hispanic whites. The same figure applies to residents of Puerto Rico. Mexican Americans are not far behind, being 1.7 times more at risk than non-Hispanic whites. Native Americans fare even worse— 2.2 times more likely than non-Hispanic whites, and some Native American tribes have rates as high as 50 percent. Adult Hawaiians, whether natives or of Asian or Pacific Islander descent, are more than twice as likely to have diabetes than whites. Asian Americans living in California are at slightly lower risk: 1.5 times that of non-Hispanic whites.

Surplus pounds

I know I sound like a broken record, but as with numerous other diseases, being overweight increases the odds of developing diabetes. Being overweight (a BMI above 24.9) is the biggest risk factor for Type 2 diabetes. The younger a woman is when she puts on extra pounds, the more likely it is that she will wind up as a diabetic. On the flip side, when women lose weight and keep it off, they can reduce their risk.

When overweight gives way to obesity—meaning a BMI of 30 or more—the risk rises exponentially.

As with cardiovascular disease, where a person carries weight is significant. Apple-shaped men and women, who have thick waists (what doctors call truncal obesity) are more prone to diabetes than pear-shaped folks who are heavy in the hips and buttocks.

Metabolic syndrome

Metabolic syndrome is composed of five risk factors that dramatically increase the likelihood of developing diabetes, as well as coronary artery disease, stroke and hypertension. Each condition is in itself a risk for diabetes and cardiovascular disease, but together they vastly compound the likelihood of serious disease. You need have only three of these five conditions to be diagnosed with metabolic syndrome:

- Truncal obesity. In men, this means a waist of 40 inches or more; in women, 35 inches or more.

- Hypertension, meaning blood pressure of 135/85 mmHg or higher.

- High triglycerides, meaning 150 mg/dL or more.

- Low HDL ("good") cholesterol, meaning less than 40 mg/dL for men and less than 50 mg/dL for women.

- High fasting blood sugar, meaning 110 mg/dL or higher.

About 44 percent of Americans over the age of 50 have metabolic syndrome, also known as prediabetes.

For women only

Two conditions associated with the female reproductive system are also linked to the development of diabetes. If a woman has had what is called gestational diabetes during pregnancy (a unique type of diabetes that goes away after she gives birth) or has given birth to an infant who weighed more than nine pounds, she has a greater likelihood of later developing Type 2 diabetes.

Likewise, women with polycystic ovary syndrome (PCOS) have an elevated risk. PCOS is a hormonal imbalance associated with insulin resistance and high levels of insulin in the blood similar to the early stages of diabetes that afflicts up to 10 percent of all women in their childbearing years. It results in enlarged ovaries, irregular menstrual periods, failure to ovulate, weight gain, infertility and excessive body hair due to excessive testosterone levels. About 35 percent of women with PCOS go on to have diabetes and typically the disease progresses much more quickly to those painful side effects than it does in women without PCOS.

In my practice, I see a low-carbohydrate diet protocol will often lead to increased fertility.

The danger of inactivity

Although you can be overweight and still be physically active, inactivity is often a contributing factor to being overweight or obese. Exercise not only helps you maintain your healthy weight or weight loss, it also increases the ratio of muscle to fat in your body. The more muscle mass you have, the higher your metabolism, which helps you burn more glucose and body fat. Also, importantly, the more muscle you have, the more responsive your body is to the effects of insulin. In fact, a review of 14 studies has shown that even without significant weight loss, moderate exercise alone improves blood sugar control. Regular vigorous exercise works on multiple levels to reduce your risk for developing diabetes.

The role of the environment

A significant body of research links two toxins—arsenic and dioxins—to increased risk for diabetes. Pesticides, toxic chemicals and a form of vitamin E were associated with a higher likelihood of Type 2 diabetes. If you have been diagnosed with elevated blood sugar or diabetes, it might be worth looking into your toxic chemical load.

Arsenic assault

Although arsenic is present in the environment in many forms, the primary way in which the general public is exposed to this poison is through contaminated drinking water. People are also exposed to arsenic in medicines to treat conditions as diverse as psoriasis and leukemia, as well as in some wines (likely via arsenic-laced pesticides) and mineral waters. Recent reports even suggest that all kinds of rice have unacceptable levels of arsenic, possibly because of high levels of arsenic in soils, whether naturally occurring or not.

Individuals who work in certain occupations (processing metal ores, manufacturing glass or pharmaceuticals and producing or applying pesticides, for example) are at heightened risk. Several research studies have shown an association between exposure to arsenic and increased risk of developing diabetes.

Deadly dioxin

The term dioxin includes a family of highly persistent fat-soluble compounds found most commonly in foods high on the food chain such as meat and dairy products. The most toxic form of dioxin is a byproduct of manufacturing and processing industries that use chlorine compounds. These include paper pulp mills, water and waste processors and manufacturers of pesticides and polyvinyl chloride (PVC) products. Dioxins also are spewed into the environment when chlorinated wastes are incinerated. In addition to a long list of health effects resulting from exposure to dioxins, high concentrations may alter glucose metabolism and hormone levels.

Although the results of research have not been consistent, several findings suggest that dioxin exposure raises the risks for developing diabetes. Research shows that men who were involved in aerial spraying of herbicides, including Agent Orange, were more likely to have diabetes, impaired glucose metabolism and impaired insulin production.

CHAPTER 13

The Importance of Diet

Talking about diabetes without discussing diet is like trying to put together a meal without any food. But I did want you to understand both the long progression to diabetes and other factors that influence whether this disease threatens your future before I get to the meat of the matter, so to speak.

First of all, let me repeat: a proper diet will prevent diabetes. Even if you already have disturbed blood sugar and insulin resistance, you can stop them in their tracks without drugs, simply by changing the way you eat. This applies even if your parents and/or siblings have Type 2 diabetes.

The way of eating I advocate is not what the American Diabetes Association (ADA) recommends. Rather, instead of obsessing about fat and allowing plenty of sugar, white flour and other nutritionally deficient foods as the ADA program does, my Fight Fat with Fat Diet approach is derived from the work of Dr. Robert C. Atkins.

Although Dr. Atkins' low-carbohydrate diet is best known for its weight-loss results, eating only fiber- and nutrient-rich carbohydrates—and avoiding processed carbohydrates—in combination with a mix of protein sources and natural fats is ideally suited to managing blood sugar and insulin levels. At the same time, this way of eating makes it easy to keep weight under control, which is, of course, also key to avoiding diabetes.

In fact, at the time of his death, Dr. Atkins was at work on the book he felt was the culmination of his life's work. *Atkins Diabetes Revolution: The Groundbreaking Approach to Preventing and Controlling Type 2 Diabetes* (Morrow, 2004) was published posthumously. Much of the book is based upon his observations from working with thousands of patients (some of whom have since become my patients) who were able to correct their metabolic disorders by changing their diet, becoming physically active and following a supplement protocol similar to the one I will describe later in this chapter.

This book is, of course, about prevention, so my focus is on how carbohydrate control effectively prevents diabetes.

Why low fat doesn't work

Everyone agrees that keeping weight down reduces the risk of developing diabetes as well as heart disease and a host of other conditions discussed in this book. Long term, the best way to control your weight is to develop healthful eating habits and eat moderately. Do that, and unless you have a major metabolic disorder or you are extremely inactive, you will arrive at a weight that is appropriate for your age and body type. But if a diet—and I am speaking of a way of eating, not specifically a weight-loss diet—is impossible to maintain because it lacks flavor and leaves you hungry and craving certain foods, it is only a matter of time before it becomes a former diet. In the decades since the American government has advocated a low-fat diet, the obesity epidemic has flowered.

Low fat is high carb

A low-fat diet, by definition, is inherently a high carbohydrate diet. That's because when you restrict fat you are restricting protein as well, since meat, poultry, fish, cheese and most other forms of protein contain good amounts of fat. What you are left with are carbohydrates, which encompasses an array of foods. Most foods contain some combination of fat, protein and carbohydrate. For example, dairy products contain carbohydrate along with fat and protein.

Low-glycemic ("good") carbohydrates are typically whole foods like leafy green vegetables, brown rice, lentils, raspberries, and hundreds of other vegetables, fruits and whole grains. Then

---

THE SAD (STANDARD AMERICAN DIET) RECIPE FOR DISASTER

When you indulge in high-glycemic refined carbohydrate foods, your blood sugar quickly rises, prompting your pancreas to release insulin to ferry the blood sugar to your cells. If you continue to eat this way, over time the cells become increasingly resistant to the effects of insulin, stimulating the pancreas to produce even more insulin. When the insulin finally kicks in, your blood sugar level dips so low that it can stimulate stress hormones that cause hunger and cravings for sweets and other simple carbs. When you give into those cravings, the cycle repeats itself and the pounds pile on.

It is these cravings that distinguish the condition known as carbohydrate addiction, which makes it so difficult for some people to take control of their weight. For example, a substances called amylopectin-A, found in all products that contain wheat, have been shown to cross the blood-brain barrier and activate the brain's opiate receptors—the same ones that respond with addictive behavior when they are exposed to morphine and other opiate drugs.

In addition to prompting the storage of excess glucose as body fat, the release of insulin has another dangerous result. The fat is transported around your body in the bloodstream in the form of triglycerides. High triglycerides, you will recall, is an independent risk factor for diabetes as well as heart disease and stroke.

there is the endless array of high-glycemic ("bad") carbs that beckon from the supermarket shelves, including the processed, refined offerings such as cookies, chips, syrupy drinks, white bread and so on.

By definition, high glycemic foods have a dramatic impact on blood sugar levels within a couple of hours after consumption. In contrast, low glycemic foods raise blood sugar levels more slowly and moderately, allowing the body's natural production of insulin to "catch up" and keep blood sugar levels off the roller coaster.

Carbs, blood sugar and insulin

While it is definitely possible to eat a high carbohydrate diet composed primarily of fresh vegetables, whole grains and fruits—witness Mediterranean cuisine—with a modest amount of fish, cheese and meat, in the U.S., a so-called low-fat diet is usually packed with high-glycemic carbs. For anyone with a genetic propensity to diabetes, that is a recipe for disaster.

Most fats are fine

When you control carbohydrates, you don't have to keep track of how much fat you are eating. The exception is trans fats, known as hydrogenated or partially hydrogenated oils, which are to be avoided at all costs. That means that you can enjoy a lamb chop, salmon, olive oil on your vegetables and in your salad dressing then whipped cream on fresh raspberries without feeling guilty. In fact, all these fats carry flavor, which makes food more satisfying. When you eliminate most fat from your diet, you yearn for flavor, which can often lead to overeating. Fats also provide a comforting satiety in a way that carbohydrates don't. By the way, eating fats with carbohydrates moderates their glycemic impact.

CHAPTER 14

The Salerno Solution Diabetes Supplement Program

A good supplement program acts as an insurance policy, even when you follow a healthful diet. The following supplements promote the metabolism of carbohydrates, improve insulin sensitivity, lower triglycerides and act as anti-inflammatories.

As I always recommend, discuss these recommendations with your health care provider to determine which are best for you and your condition.

Biotin

A water-soluble B vitamin, also known as vitamin H, biotin is key to the metabolism of energy, enabling four essential enzymes to break down carbohydrates into glucose, fats into fatty acids and protein into amino acids. Produced in the body by certain types of intestinal bacteria, biotin is also found in foods such as brewer's yeast, nutritional yeast, oat bran, whole grains, nuts and nut butters, egg yolks, sardines, legumes, liver and other organ meats, bananas, cauliflower and mushrooms.

People with Type 2 diabetes often are deficient in biotin. Long-term use of antibiotics can also depress biotin levels.

Optimal daily dose: 2–4 mg. *Note:* Biotin appears to work synergistically with chromium to control blood sugar, so be sure to take the two supplements together.

Chromium

Like biotin, the trace mineral chromium plays a role in the metabolism of carbohydrates, protein and fat, helping your body to metabolize fat, turn protein into muscle and convert carbohydrate into energy. Chromium is necessary to make glucose tolerance factor, which enhances the action of insulin, facilitating the process by which glucose is transported to the liver, muscle and fat cells. There it can be converted for energy as needed, keeping blood sugar levels under control. Deficiency in chromium results in impaired glucose tolerance, insulin resistance and diabetes-like symptoms. In addition, chromium acts as an appetite suppressant.

Chromium supplements have also been shown to improve glucose tolerance and reduce abnormally high blood levels of insulin in pregnant women with gestational diabetes. Since heart disease is often a complication of diabetes, improvements in cholesterol and triglycerides are valuable benefits.

Vigorous exercise can deplete the body's stores of chromium. Processing foods also depletes them of most of the trace minerals. Trace amounts of chromium are found in many foods, among them brewer's yeast, beef, cheese, leafy dark greens, mushrooms, shellfish and barley.

Optimal daily dose: 200–600 mg. *Note:* Chromium should be taken with biotin for maximum effectiveness. Look for chromium in its nicotinate form, which is most absorbable.

Vanadium

Along with biotin and chromium, vanadium helps get the proper amounts of glucose into the body's cells. This trace mineral is found in black pepper, mushrooms, sunflower and safflower seeds and oil, olive oil, shellfish, parsley, dill seed, buckwheat, oats, rice, green beans, carrots, cabbage, radishes and eggs. *In vivo* and *in vitro* studies have shown that vanadium mimics the effects of insulin.

Vanadium can lower blood sugar levels and improve sensitivity to insulin in both Type 1 and Type 2 diabetes.

In parts of the world where vanadium (and selenium) soil levels are high, there are lower than average rates of heart disease. Nonetheless, too much vanadium can be dangerous.

Optimal daily dose: 30–60 mg vanadyl sulfate or 1–2 mg vanadyl. *Note:* Excessive levels of vanadyl can be toxic so be sure not to exceed dosage.

Coenzyme Q-10 (Co Q-10)

This essential micronutrient, produced by the body, is important for dozens of body functions, but production slows with age. Co Q-10 plays an important role in producing energy for the mitochondria found in every cell in your body. People with diabetes typically have lower levels of Co Q-10 than healthy people. If you are taking statin drugs, Co Q-10 supplementation is essential since the drug depletes your body's natural production.

Optimal daily dose: 100–300 mg

Alpha lipoic acid

The antioxidant alpha lipoic acid assists the body in using glucose, which enables it to improve blood sugar control. In one study, people with Type 2 diabetes who were given intravenous supplemental alpha lipoic acid (ALA) saw an increase in insulin release and a reduction in blood sugar levels.

One way in which antioxidants, of which ALA is one, help fight diabetes is by neutralizing free radicals in your body involved in the development of insulin resistance. Supplementing with ALA has been shown to enhance uptake of glucose by tissues.

Diabetic neuropathy is a nerve damage complication of diabetes, which results in pain, tingling and numbness in the extremities. It can be relieved with supplemental ALA. One study showed that nerve function was restored after four months on high oral doses. ALA improves nerve blood flow, reduces oxidative stress and improves nerve function.

Optimal daily dose: 600–1,000 mg

N-acetyl cysteine

N-acetyl cysteine (NAC) is a form of the amino acid cysteine, which helps the body synthesize the antioxidant glutathione that has been shown to improve insulin sensitivity. When insulin levels are high, free radicals flourish, which can destroy various types of tissue.

Optimal daily dose: 1–2 mg. *Note:* NAC should be accompanied by 15 mg of zinc and 2 mg of copper per day.

Gymnema sylvestre

Also known as Gurmar and Meshashringi, the leaves of the plant *gymnema sylvestre* have been used for centuries in Ayurvedic medicine to regulate glucose metabolism. In fact, the Hindi name gurmar translates as "sugar destroyer." Unlike a prescription drug, *gymnema* lowers blood sugar levels gradually by helping regenerate the ability of the pancreas to produce insulin, thus helping balance blood sugar levels. (Unlike insulin and other drugs, *gymnema* won't lower blood sugar to dangerous levels). It also interferes with glucose absorption in the intestine, which helps keep the pancreas from releasing too much insulin. The herb also helps the uptake of glucose by the cells and keeps adrenaline from stimulating the liver to produce glucose. Finally, it banishes the taste of sugar, which suppresses cravings for sweets, making it easier to lose weight.

Optimal daily dose: 200 mg

Banaba leaf extract

Long used in the Philippines as a natural plant insulin for blood sugar control, banaba leaf appears to balance blood sugar by promoting healthy insulin levels and stimulating the transport of glucose into cells. It also is said to help control cravings, particularly for carbohydrates, and may promote weight loss.

In a clinical study of people with Type 2 diabetes who received a standardized extract of banaba leaf that contained one percent corosolic acids showed a 30 percent decrease in blood sugar levels after two weeks.

Optimal daily dose: 50 mg

Cinnamon

Next time you sprinkle cinnamon on your cappuccino or your oatmeal, you may also be cutting your risk for diabetes and cardiovascular disease. The familiar spice is a potent antioxidant with the potential to help maintain healthy blood sugar and cholesterol levels. The Chinese used cinnamon for an array of medical complaints ranging from diarrhea to influenza as long as 4,000 years ago. It was also used, as many spices were, to preserve food in the days before refrigeration.

Regular supplementation with cinnamon may be able to reduce fasting blood sugar, triglycerides, LDL cholesterol and total cholesterol.

Optimal daily dose: 125–250 mg

Magnesium

Magnesium lowers blood glucose levels, increases insulin sensitivity and calms the sympathetic nervous system.

Although the relationship between magnesium and diabetes has been studied for decades, it is still poorly understood.

However, what is known about diabetes and magnesium embodies a persuasive list encouraging supplementation:

- Low magnesium levels are common findings in non-insulin-dependent diabetic patients. In fact, diabetes is a frequent cause of secondary hypomagnesemia (lower blood levels of magnesium). Poorly controlled diabetics excrete more magnesium than do nondiabetics. Magnesium assists in the maintenance of the pancreatic cells that produce insulin. Scientists believe that a magnesium deficiency interrupts insulin secretion and its activity. Magnesium, by enhancing the action of insulin, improves insulin's ability to transport glucose into the cells.

- Magnesium increases the number and sensitivity of insulin receptors.

- An increase in red blood cell magnesium significantly and positively correlated with an increase in both insulin secretion and action.

- As magnesium levels plummet, the incidence of diabetic complications escalates, especially those that are heart-related.

- Magnesium is the mineral of choice to reduce hyperresponsiveness in the sympathetic nervous system (SNS). This is important to people with diabetes because when the SNS is alerted, blood glucose levels tend to be higher. Since diabetes is aggravated by stress, magnesium supplementation may help you find an inner calm.

In Conclusion

Diabetes mellitus is a disease that causes your body to be unable to quickly and efficiently deal with blood sugar (glucose) produced from the breakdown of carbohydrates and other foods by insulin, which is created by the pancreas. There are two types:

Type 1, also known as juvenile diabetes, most commonly appears in children, adolescents and young adults and is a result of a malfunctioning pancreas. Type 2, which until recently was called adult-onset diabetes, results from a pancreas that has been exhausted by a lifestyle of poor diet and lack of exercise, which creates a situation where the pancreas makes insulin, but the insulin does not work as it should.

In a nutshell, these are ways to prevent or reduce the possibility of developing diabetes:

• Exercise at least a half-hour most days of the week.

• Focus on eating fiber- and nutrient-rich complex carbohydrates and avoid processed carbohydrates. Combine these with a mix of healthy protein sources and natural fats to manage blood sugar and insulin levels.

• Follow a good supplement program that promotes the metabolism of carbohydrates, improves insulin sensitivity, lowers triglycerides and acts to reduce inflammation.

Diabetes is the fourth leading cause of death by disease globally. At least 50 percent of all people with diabetes are unaware of their condition. In some countries this figure may reach 80 percent.

In addition to diabetes, the condition of impaired glucose tolerance (IGT), in which the blood glucose level is higher than normal but not as high as in diabetes, is also a major public health problem. People with IGT have a higher risk of developing diabetes as well as an increased risk of cardiovascular disease.

Cancer

CHAPTER 15

Basic Cancer Prevention

Before we begin to talk about how to combat cancer, let's understand the enemy we are fighting.

Cancer is created by a series of complex events in the human body. For undetermined reasons, some genetic and some environmental, cells begin to reproduce wildly, abnormally lengthening their natural lifespan, and creating tumors. This process, known medically as apoptosis, creates rogue cells that refuse to die. Then these rogue cells are carried to other parts of the body, either by blood vessels or the lymphatic system, spreading (or metastasizing) these cancerous cells to other parts of the body.

Tragically, cancer of all types is slowly approaching heart disease as the number one killer worldwide. It is estimated that over 1.6 million new cases of cancer will be diagnosed in 2013. Aside from nonmelanoma skin cancers, breast and prostate cancers are the most frequently diagnosed cancers in women and men, respectively, followed by lung and colorectal cancers in both men and women.

And despite billions spent on research, the cancer death rate decreased only slightly from 1950 to 2003, while rates for other major chronic diseases decreased substantially during this period. The cure rates for nearly all cancers are similar today to what they were 50 years ago, but survival time has improved, thanks to the technological advances and screenings that lead to early detection.

Finally, certain forms of cancer, especially prostate, breast, skin and thyroid, have been on the rise in recent decades. Many of these diagnoses are the direct result of increases in the number of people being screened as well as improvements in screening technology.

The sad truth is that we are not making progress toward a cure for cancer. Our best hope is to find ways to prevent cancer, since it is clear that at least half of all cancer deaths can be prevented.

The good news

There are many facets to cancer prevention: a good diet, weight control and physical activity, a healthy environment, avoidance of carcinogens such as those in tobacco smoke, and screening of populations at risk to allow early detection. The use of food and nutrients as protection from cancer makes sense because of their long-standing use, their relative lack of toxicity, and recent encouraging research.

There is a large body of research on nutrients that have been shown to significantly reduce the risk of numerous cancers. Many are powerful antioxidants that can suppress free radicals in the body. Some fortify the immune system, allowing it to fight off disease before it gains a foothold. Others act as anti-inflammatories, making the body less susceptible to disease. Still others are natural antibiotics.

CHAPTER 16

The Salerno Solution Basic Cancer Supplement Program

H ere is a baker's dozen of nutrients, all of them supported with solid research, that belong in your arsenal of cancer-fighting weapons. Each includes an optimal daily dose, which reflects the daily requirement or Recommended Daily Allowance (RDA) for adults. As always, discuss with your doctor which of these will work best for your individual situation.

A multi-vitamin with folic acid

I recommend a multi-vitamin for everyone, but for those who have a particular focus on cancer prevention, look for one that contains folic acid. Folic acid, one of the B vitamins, occurs naturally in the form of folate in leafy dark greens such as spinach and kale as well as beans, beets and corn, citrus fruits and most berries. It also occurs in organ meats. But most people do not eat enough of these foods. Moreover, cooking destroys most of the folic acid. Finally, folic acid needs to be consumed with vitamins B_{12} and B_6 to be effective. The best way to ensure adequate intake of this crucial nutrient is as part of a multi-vitamin.

Folic acid deficiency is known to be associated with a dramatic increase in a pregnant woman's risk of delivering a baby with spinal bifida or other neural tube defects. As a result, all women of childbearing age are advised to take a multi-vitamin that contains 400 micrograms of folic acid.

Preventing life-shattering birth defects is only part of the power of this important nutrient. It also is a powerful anticarcinogen. A study at Harvard Medical School of 88,756 female nurses that began in 1980 showed that women who took a comprehensive multi-vitamin with 400 micrograms or more of folic acid daily for more than 15 years were 45 percent less likely to develop colon cancer and 20 percent less likely to develop any form of cancer than women whose daily intake was 200 micrograms or less each day. Other studies have shown similar benefits in reducing colon cancer risk for men.

Optimal daily dose: 800 mcg

Selenium

Selenium, a trace mineral found in the soil, combines with proteins to function as an antioxidant. Although it is essential to eat plenty of vegetables and fruits to maintain good health, in many parts of the world the soil is depleted of nutrients, including selenium, making supplementation of this nutrient essential.

This trace mineral is well known as a cancer fighter. A famous study on the role of selenium in protecting against skin cancer found no positive correlation for skin cancer. However, men and women who had taken selenium supplements (200 micrograms) for 10 years had significantly lower risks for several other cancers, including colorectal cancer, than those taking a placebo.

A more recent study that pooled results from three clinical studies comprising 1,700 patients who had had surgery on cancerous polyps in the colon confirmed that selenium is effective at combating colorectal cancer. The researchers checked the selenium blood levels of all the patients and found that those with the highest levels had a 34 percent reduction in colon cancer recurrence than those with the lowest levels.

As with many other forms of cancer, individuals with lung cancer have been found to have low levels of selenium. I will discuss this study again in a future chapter, but its results in the case of lung cancer prevention are so dramatic, it is worth repeating. A carefully constructed study of individuals with a history of skin cancer was set up to see if treating them with selenium would improve their outcome. Although whether the subjects received selenium or a placebo over the four-and-a-half year period of the study had no apparent effect on skin cancer, researchers found that the nutrient did cut the risk of developing several other forms of cancer by 37 percent and cut deaths from cancer by 50 percent. In the case of lung cancer, there was a 46 percent decrease in the incidence of lung cancer and a 53 percent decrease in deaths from it.

A major clinical study funded by the National Cancer Institute yielded encouraging results showing indications that selenium added cancer preventive agents and altered lung cancer cells. And while we don't fully understand how this works, it is encouraging nonetheless.

Optimal daily dose: 200 mcg

Zinc

Like selenium, zinc is an essential trace mineral and is the second most abundant trace mineral in the body (after iron). Zinc plays a major role in the immune system and is also an antioxidant. Oysters are the richest source of zinc. Red meat, poultry, certain cheeses, shrimp, crab, and other shellfish are also good sources. Zinc is better absorbed in the presence of protein, so zinc in plant sources (such as lima beans, pinto beans, soybeans, peanuts and other legumes, whole grains, miso, tofu, brewer's yeast, cooked greens, mushrooms, tahini and pumpkin and sunflower seeds) is less easily absorbed.

Like selenium, the soil's concentrations of zinc have been depleted. Today's soil contains 60 percent less of the mineral than it did 50 years ago. Taking zinc supplements is vitally important, as a deficiency can result in a host of medical problems.

Zinc supplementation is associated with a 45 percent decrease in the risk of prostate cancer in men using zinc supplements daily.

Optimal daily dose: 50 mg

Soy

The risks of postmenopausal breast cancer were lower among women with high intakes of soy and isoflavone (a compound found in soy), although even moderate intake showed protective benefits. These results suggested that soy and isoflavone food intake has a protective effect on postmenopausal breast cancer. However, studies have not shown such a protective characteristic of soy among premenopausal women.

Fermented soy milk, miso, natte and tempeh or dietary supplements are the best sources.

Optimal daily dose: 100 mg

Fish Oils

Well known for their cardiovascular and other benefits, fish oils are a basic essential nutrient, which are also valuable for reducing the risk of cancer. In a well-designed 1999 study on fish oil, men who ate fish three times a week or consumed fish oil supplements daily were 30 percent less likely to develop prostate cancer and 50 percent less likely to die from any form of cancer.

A review of laboratory, animal and population-based studies points strongly toward the advisability of consuming a diet high in omega-3 fatty acids as a deterrent to colorectal cancer. For example, consuming as little as 2.5 grams of fish oils daily has been found effective in preventing the progression from benign polyps to colon cancer. In the U.S. and other westernized countries, the typical diet includes a ratio of omega-6s to omega-3s of 20:1. The ideal for good health and disease prevention is actually 2:1.

Like aspirin and other NSAIDs, fish oil works as an anti-inflammatory, which may mean that part of its effectiveness against the development of cancer is that it blocks the development of prostaglandins that can inflame the colon and lay the foundation for cancer at a later date.

Researchers suggest that eating fish reduces the risk of developing cancer, including lung cancer, because certain cold-water fatty fish are high in omega-3 fatty acids. Since very few people eat fish five times a week and I certainly don't advise such heavy consumption because of the risk of heavy-metal contamination from mercury, fish oil supplements are an excellent way to get omega-3 fatty acids on a regular basis.

Optimal daily dose: 1,000–2,000 mg *Note:* Use caution if taking blood thinners and reduce dose accordingly.

Diidolylmethane (DIM)/Indole-3-Carbinol

This pair of nutrients found in cabbage, broccoli, cauliflower and other cruciferous vegetables have been shown to reduce the risk of contracting lung, stomach, colon, breast and rectal cancers by more than 50 percent.

Optimal daily dose: 200 mg

Vitamin E

Vitamin E is a fat-soluble vitamin found in foods such as vegetable oils, wheat germ, whole grains, almonds, hazelnuts, peanut butter and sunflower seeds. For 60 years, researchers have been studying the immune-system boosting role of this powerful antioxidant in defending the body against free radicals and thereby inhibiting malignancies. A study published in 2000 demonstrated that a daily vitamin E intake of 400 IU reduced prostate and bladder cancer risk by more 30 percent after 12 years.

Any nutrients that can repair damaged DNA or protect it from damage theoretically might reduce the incidence of lung cancer, in which damaging oxidants are taken into the lungs. As with some other antioxidants, researchers have found that individuals who have high levels of vitamin E in their blood are less likely to develop lung cancer than those with lower levels. Likewise, individuals whose diet is higher in foods that contain vitamin E are less likely to develop the disease than those deficient in dietary vitamin E.

It turns out that researchers on the benefits of vitamin E may have been barking up the wrong tree, metaphorically, or were barking up only one tree instead of several. There are actually seven different forms of vitamin E, but most manufactured supplements contain only alpha-tocopherol, but not gamma-tocopherol, which is the form found in corn, walnuts, pecans, sesame seeds and some other grains, seeds and nuts. Studies have shown that gamma–tocopherol in combination with delta-tocopherol inhibits the growth and induces death of human lung cancer and prostate cancer cells. Normal cells were not damaged.

When taking vitamin E as a supplement, be sure to use the naturally occurring form of alpha-tocopherol with gamma-tocopherol.

Optimal daily dose: 800 IU. *Note:* Use caution if using blood thinners and reduce dose accordingly.

Green Tea

Another powerful antioxidant, green tea protects liver cells and spurs the immune system into action. Research in Russia has shown that the antioxidants in green tea offer protection against toxins in alcohol and cigarette smoke. Drinking more than 10 cups of green tea a day is associated with healthy liver function. Green tea also removes excess iron from the bloodstream.

Green tea, long a dietary staple in Japan, has recently become a "hot" nutrient in the Western world, and for good reason. Green tea contains four antioxidants, including the powerful epigallocatechin gallate (EGCG). Many studies have shown that consuming green tea reduces the risk of developing cancer. People who live in Uji and Shizuoka, which produce most of the green tea in Japan, are reputed to have among the lowest rates of cancer in the world. A study published in 2000 revealed that subjects who consumed more than 10 cups of green tea daily cut their risk of all forms of cancer by nearly 50 percent. For those who do not want to consume that much caffeine, this invaluable antioxidant is available as a pure extract.

Green tea has many cancer-protective mechanisms, including antioxidant properties, the ability to arrest the division of mutant cells, and the ability to cause cells to die. White tea, which is even less processed than green tea and has higher levels of polyphenols and antioxidants, is also attracting interest as a component of a healthy diet.

Several studies, mostly done in Asia, where green tea is much more commonly consumed than in the West, show a correlation between increased consumption of the beverage and reduction in the risk for colorectal cancer. The more green tea individuals drink, the less their likelihood of getting colon cancer.

A study at the Linus Pauling Institute at the Oregon State University, which has been in the forefront of green tea research, provided provocative results that could point to disease prevention for humans. The researchers used laboratory mice that are genetically predisposed to cancer (particularly of the intestinal tract). The study demonstrated that green (and white) teas are as effective as the prescription NSAID Sulindac, commonly used to prevent certain colon cancers. (Sulindac typically reduces tumor formation by about 50 percent.) One group of mice was fed green tea, another white tea; a control group was given no treatment at all. Still others were given either green or white tea in combination with Sulindac. The mice that got nothing developed an average of about 30 tumors each. The mice that drank green tea had an average of 17 tumors each; those that drank white tea got an average of 13 tumors. The most dramatic results came from mice that were given both Sulindac *and* white tea: each averaged six tumors.

If the results of this study can be replicated in humans, it suggests that a combination of green or white tea with an NSAID could dramatically reduce the risk for certain cancers of the colon.

Despite the dramatic results that regular and heavy aspirin use has shown in reducing the risk of advanced colon cancer, the side effects, including gastric bleeding and ulcers, can be serious. So another promising aspect of this study is that it suggests that smaller doses of aspirin or another drug could be equally effective in combination with tea. And those who cannot tolerate NSAIDs at all could get the same protection the drugs afford without the dangerous side effects.

Optimal daily dose: as a supplement: 200 mg *Note:* Use caution with green tea if you are taking blood thinners like Coumadin because it can thin blood to dangerous levels.

Garlic

An edible member of the lily family, garlic is not just a culinary star. Thanks to its allyl sulfur compounds, garlic is also a therapeutic wonder that slows or prevents the growth of tumor cells, among numerous other benefits. Garlic has been shown to reduce the risk of stomach and colorectal cancer by up to 40 percent, according to a study done in 2000 that indicates that more than 20 grams or five cloves per week is optimal. Garlic supplements provide the same benefits without the bitter aftertaste, garlic breath or gastrointestinal side effects.

There has been considerable research on whether eating a lot of garlic is associated with a lower risk of developing colorectal cancer. Organosulfur compounds are formed when you cut or crush garlic, and they are associated with disease prevention and treatment. A meta-analysis of six studies found that people who ate the most garlic were about 30 percent less likely to get colorectal cancer than those who ate the least. One form of garlic apparently even has the ability to suppress the growth and progression of polyps that have already formed in the colon and rectum, effectively halting the possible progression toward cancer.

In a recent Japanese study, 37 patients who were found to have colorectal polyps during a colonoscopy were divided into two groups. Some were treated with a large dose of aged garlic extract (AGE); the others were treated with a very low dose. Neither patients nor researchers knew who was getting what dose. Before starting the AGE therapy, all polyps over a certain size were removed and any small remaining polyps were measured. After six and 12 months, colonoscopies were repeated. At a year, those individuals who had a very low dose of AGE had developed more polyps, but in the high-dose group both the size and the number of polyps were significantly reduced.

Optimal daily dose: 400 mg (Eat as much raw garlic as you like.)

Olive Oil

Another food better known for its cardiovascular benefits, olive oil has anti-inflammatory and antioxidant properties that make it a valuable weapon in the anticancer arsenal. A 2011 study concluded that olive oil has a protective role against breast and stomach cancers. Olive oil has also shown benefits with other forms of cancer, including colon and ovarian. Whether you dress salad and other vegetables with olive oil or take it in supplemental form, be sure to use olive oil on a daily basis. Extra virgin olive oil is preferable over other forms.

Optimal daily dose: 200 mg

Resveratrol (Red Wine Extract)

This potent antioxidant found in grape skins, peanuts and other plants stimulates Phase II metabolizing enzymes that detoxify poisons, including carcinogens. It also encourages apoptosis, the natural death of cancer cells, inhibiting the progression to full-blown cancer. In the case of liver cancer, resveratrol also seems to inhibit the rapid growth of cells and block the invasive properties of tumor cells.

Resveratrol is both a plant antibiotic and an antioxidant. The skins of certain wine grapes are the most abundant source of the nutrient. The longer the skins remain in the fermentation process, the higher the resveratrol content, which is why red wine is a significantly better source than white.

A study published in 2000 reported that individuals who drank one to two glasses of red wine each day reduced their overall cancer risk by 20 percent compared to non-drinkers.

Optimal daily dose: 500 mg

Vitamin A/Carotene

Fruits and vegetables that are a rich source of carotenoids (including squashes, sweet potatoes, tomatoes and red and yellow bell peppers) are thought to provide health benefits by decreasing the risk of various diseases, particularly certain cancers. In part, the beneficial effects of carotenoids are thought to be due to their role as antioxidants.

Some observational studies have also shown these carotenoids may help reduce the risk of certain types of cancer, particularly those of the breast and lung.

Optimal daily dose: 10,000 units

Turmeric

A key ingredient in curry powder (and what supplies its golden hue), turmeric has been shown to inhibit carcinogens, to increase the body's production of glutathione (a potent cancer-fighter), and to promote the liver's ability to detoxify potential carcinogens. Turmeric is also an anti-inflammatory.

Curcumin, the agent most responsible for most of the biological activity of turmeric, is more easily absorbed into the body. Curcumin, a flavonoid, is well documented as an anti-inflammatory, antioxidant and anticarcinogen. Curcumin inhibits production of the compound thromboxane, which the body produces in response to inflammation. However, thromboxane can overdo its job, causing blood vessels to constrict and actually increase inflammation. Curcumin does not inhibit prostacyclin, which responds to inflammation in a more measured and appropriate fashion. In the test tube, curcumin has been shown to inhibit the mutation of cells by tobacco smoke. This finding suggests that curcumin could help protect the lining of cells from the effects of smoking.

Optimal daily dose: 400–1,000 mg

Coenzyme Q-10 (Co Q-10)

This important tool for overall body health also has a role on cancer prevention. Our bodies use the antioxidant coenzyme Q-10 (CoQ-10) to quash free radicals throughout the body and to defend and mend cellular DNA. Although Co Q-10 is found in most of the body's tissues, the lowest amounts are found in the lungs. Low blood levels of Co Q-10 have been found in patients with lung cancer, as well as many other forms of cancer.

The liver and the antioxidant Co Q-10 are intimately en-twined. Foods supply coenzyme Q-3, -4 or –5, which the liver transforms to Q-10, which in turn is transformed into adenosine triphosphate (ATP), the form of energy that powers our bodies. Once ATP is released into the blood stream, it travels to virtually every cell in the body. Co Q-10 is also known as ubiquitone, because it is ubiquitous—or everywhere—in the body, although the heart and the liver contain the most. As we age, our bodies produce smaller amounts of Co Q-10 and studies have shown that when people die of organ failure, their bodies are deficient in Co Q-10. The nutrient has been shown to restore liver function after damage to the organ. *Optimal daily dose:* 100–200 mg. *Note:* Take with meals for best absorption and ask for medical guidance if you are taking blood thinners.

Vitamin D

Another everybody-needs-it nutrient that is part of our basic list is important in cancer prevention. Our bodies produce vitamin D primarily through exposure to sunlight. While a moderate exposure to sunlight is good for us, too much can cause skin cancers and too little can foster other types of cancer. So moderation is the key here.

Vitamin D and calcium belong to a mutual admiration society: the body requires sufficient stores of vitamin D in order to absorb calcium. That's why vitamin D is so important in helping prevent osteoporosis among the elderly. It also appears to be an ally in protecting your body against several cancers, including colorectal cancer. A number of studies have shown benefits in reducing colorectal cancer risk when vitamin D is combined with calcium, vitamin E, selenium and other nutrients. But vitamin D appears to have protective effects independent of other nutrients, including calcium.

One review study looked at earlier studies of vitamin D and colon cancer conducted between 1966 and 2004, some of which measured dietary and supplement intake and others (which could come also from sunlight) measured blood levels. Ten of 18 studies found that individuals who did not get adequate vitamin D had a higher risk of developing colon cancer. The authors suggested that daily intake of 1,000 IU of vitamin D cut colon cancer risk by about 50 percent.

Good dietary sources of vitamin D include oily fish such as

salmon and sardines as well as fortified milk. Other foods like orange juice and yogurt are often fortified as well, but it can still be hard to get enough without taking supplements.

If you live in a southern clime, just a few minutes in the sun several days a week gives you plenty of vitamin D. (Of course, you need to protect yourself from too much sun.) But if you live north of 40 degrees latitude (north of Denver, for example) for about half the year you won't get enough sun for your body to convert it to vitamin D. In fact, people in certain parts of the

BASIC CANCER SUPPLEMENT PROGRAM

Be sure to check the *Notes* in the text on those supplements with an *.

Supplement	Optimal Daily Dose
A multi-vitamin with folic acid	800 mcg
Vitamin A/Carotene	10,000 units
Vitamin E *	800 IU
Vitamin D	3,000 to 5,000 IU
Green Tea *	200 mg
Garlic	400 mg
Olive Oil	200 mg
Resveratrol (Red Wine Extract)	200 mg
Soy	100 mg
Fish Oils *	1,000–2,000 mg
Turmeric/Curcumin	400–1,000 mg
Selenium	200 mcg
Zinc	50 mg
Coenzyme Q10 (Co Q-10) *	100–200 mg
Diidolylmethane (DIM)/Indole-3-Carbinol	200 mg

world who have lower than optimal levels of vitamin D have higher rates of certain cancers. Regular supplementation ensures you have adequate levels at all times.

Optimal daily dose: 3,000 to 5,000 IU

In Conclusion

In the following chapters, as we look at how to reduce your risk of getting a variety of specific forms of cancer, we'll examine more nutrients. This list is a good general one of supplements that I advise everyone concerned with cancer to add to their menu of allies.

CHAPTER 17

Liver Cancer

The name of the largest organ inside your body is apt, because without your liver, you cannot live. The football-sized organ weighs between three to five pounds and is located below your diaphragm and above your stomach slightly on the right side of your chest. It processes and stores nutrients and regulates how much glucose, fat and protein enter your bloodstream. The liver also plays a role in helping blood clot. Finally, and importantly, the liver is key to processing and eliminating toxins, including the hormones your body produces. A well-functioning liver can banish these toxins before they harm any of your organs or systems. There are three distinct ways in which the liver detoxifies your body:

- It filters all the blood in your body, at the amazing pace of two quarts per minute.

- It secretes bile, which enables the breakdown of cholesterol, allowing toxins stored in fat and cholesterol to be neutralized and excreted.

- It breaks down and expels toxins with enzymes in a two-phase process explained below.

Although the liver is exposed to poisons, including carcinogens, on a daily basis, it is extremely resilient and can even repair or replace its own damaged tissue. This is not to say that this workhorse cannot be worked to death. The liver is subject to several diseases, some of which cause irreparable damage.

Liver cancer is primarily a lifestyle disease and is linked to, but not exclusively caused by, excess alcohol consumption, intravenous drug use, some types of sexual contact, body piercing and tattooing. Abstaining from these risky behaviors is the best way to prevent liver cancer.

Liver cancer can occur when the liver is overloaded with toxins, whether in the form of alcohol, second hand smoke, industrial chemicals, fertilizers and pesticides in food, pharmaceutical, over-the-counter and recreational drugs or any other toxins. Good nutrition and regular detoxification are essential to minimize the likelihood of most forms of cancer and many other conditions that can be life threatening. Good nutrition and regular detoxes are particularly important in the case of the liver, which bears the burden of detoxifying the entire body.

Liver cancer comes in several forms, the most common of which (in adults) is hepatocellular carcinoma (HCC), which originates in the liver's main cells. These hepatocytes perform various metabolic, endocrine and excretory functions. About 75 to 80 percent of cancers that originate in the liver are of this type. HCC is most commonly caused by cirrhosis, hepatitis and eating food contaminated with aflatoxin, all of which I'll discuss below.

The most common form of HCC in the U.S. is not a single tumor but occurs in numerous spots in the liver. It is often linked to cirrhosis of the liver caused by alcoholism and hepatitis B and C. Another form of liver cancer is cholangiocarcinoma, which originates in the liver's small bile ducts, and accounts for about 15 percent of all liver cancer. There are several other rare forms, but I will confine my discussion to the most common types.

In the U.S., it is estimated that in 2013 just over 30,000 new cases of primary liver cancer (including bile duct cancer) will be diagnosed, and just over 21,000 people will die of the disease.

Most liver cancer is secondary or metastatic, meaning it started elsewhere in the body. Primary liver cancer, which starts in the liver, accounts for only about 2 percent of cancers in the U.S., but up to half of all cancers in some undeveloped countries. This is mainly due to the prevalence of hepatitis abroad, caused by contagious viruses, that predispose a person to liver cancer. In the U.S., primary liver cancer strikes twice as many men as women at an average age of 67.

Diseases and conditions associated with liver cancer

As with other forms of cancer, liver cancer can start with damage to the DNA. Hepatitis B and C both can damage the liver, and such damage is a primary cause of hepatitis-related liver cancer. In the U.S., hepatitis C (HCV), which is transmitted through unscreened blood transfusions, contaminated needles used for injecting drugs, body piercing, or tattooing and occasionally by sexual contact, is to blame for half the cases of HCC. In the case of hepatitis B (HBV), which is spread through sexual contact and contaminated needles, a pregnant mother can pass the virus to her unborn child. The virus causes genetic changes, although of a different sort, in both cases.

Research indicates that individuals who already have HCV are less likely to develop liver cancer if given the drugs interferon and ribavirin in combination. The ribavirin/interferon combination showed improved response compared with interferon alone in patients with type 4 chronic hepatitis C without cirrhosis. However, the interferon therapies carry with them substantial health risks in themselves, including depression and irritability, extreme fatigue and flu-like symptoms, weight loss, skin rashes, gastrointestinal distress and even additional liver damage. Other drugs appear to help prevent HCV's progression to liver cancer.

Cirrhosis of the liver, usually caused by excessive alcohol consumption, can permanently scar the liver, leaving it vulnerable to cancer. Cirrhosis has been implicated in up to 80 percent of all cases of HCC. A condition known as hereditary hemochromatosis, a blood disease in which excessive deposits of iron settle in the liver and other tissues, can also cause cirrhosis.

An inflammation of the bile ducts in the liver called primary biliary cirrhosis significantly increases the risk for cholangiocarcinoma. Ulcerative colitis, the inflammation of the colon and digestive tract, and gallstones can cause changes within the bile ducts and also can lay the groundwork for this type of liver cancer. In Southeast Asia, liver parasites can contribute to developing the disease, as well.

Liver cancer can also be stimulated by exposure to industrial chemicals.

The best way to protect yourself against liver cancer is to avoid getting hepatitis, cirrhosis of the liver or other liver diseases. The wisest course of action to avoid hepatitis B and C is:

• to avoid risky behavior (including having unprotected sex with someone whose sexual history you don't know)

• do not indulge in illegal drugs

• use new needles if you must inject prescription drugs

• avoid or limit alcohol intake

• be sure to avoid certain medications that may cause liver damage, including acetaminophen (which is marketed as Tylenol, Nyquil, Theraflu, Midol and Excedrin, among other brand names) that can cause acute liver failure even at the prescribed dosages, especially in children.

• never take acetaminophen products with alcohol, a combination that multiplies the risk of liver damage.

Assessing your risks

A family history of liver cancer, including genetic mutations, increases the risk of getting the disease. As I mentioned, men are more prone to liver cancer than are women, as are people over the age of 60. Asian Americans have the highest rate of the disease in the U.S. because they have high rates of infection with hepatitis B. Less prone than Asian Americans, African Americans and Hispanics are still more likely to develop liver cancer than Caucasians.

Once again, smoking and consuming excessive amounts of alcohol (more than two drinks a day for men and one for women) increases the likelihood of developing cirrhosis, which in turn increases the likelihood of developing liver cancer. The liver turns alcohol into acetaldehyde, which is toxic to the liver.

When someone has a yeast overgrowth, commonly called a yeast infection, the yeast ferments dietary sugar (in any form), turning it into acetaldehyde, so the result is much the same as drinking too much alcohol. Moreover, the combination of yeast and sugar forms ammonia in the gut, which further damages the liver. If you have a chronic yeast overgrowth, consult your health care professional about how to change your diet to bring this condition under control.

In addition to the liver and gastrointestinal disorders discussed above, having diabetes is also linked to an increased receptivity to liver cancer. (Remember that the liver is charged with the responsibility for regulating blood sugar and converting it into glycogen, a form the body can store for a while.) An overweight person with diabetes (which many are) is also subject to a condition called fatty liver, that adds to the increased risk of liver cancer. A person with both diabetes and hepatitis C is even more at risk.

In the chapter on hormonally-related cancers, I discuss the gene mutations that predispose women to developing breast and ovarian cancer. Those same mutations, known as BRCA1 and BRCA2, have also been linked to a moderate increase in other cancers, including liver cancer. Taking birth control pills or synthetic hormone replacement therapy (HRT) also can stress the liver.

Since toxins are stored in fat, maintaining a healthy weight can help prevent toxins from accumulating in the body.

What we take into our bodies matters

It is not just the larger world of air and water pollution that threatens your liver's health. There are also seemingly innocuous substances we often put into or on our bodies without thinking much about them. I've already discussed some of these, such as consuming alcohol and using birth control pills or synthetic HRT.

Drugs—both legal and illegal

Certain drugs that are typically not problematic when used occasionally can be toxic when regularly used in large quantities. A case in point: downing eight to 12 aspirin or acetaminophen tablets or capsules a day to manage the pain of arthritis or another condition can damage the liver over time. Natural anti-inflammatories like curcumin, boswellia, strontium, willow bark, arnica and calendula can all provide safe pain relief.

Similarly, prescription drugs such as Dilantin (phenytoin) and phenobarbitol for epilepsy, antifungals Nizoral (ketoconazole) and fluoxetine for yeast overgrowth, Prilosec (omeprazole) and the tranquilizer Chlorpromazine can cause damage if used for prolonged periods at high doses.

And then there are the illegal drugs. Using anabolic steroids to bulk up muscle, which impacts your health in many ways, increases the risk of developing liver cancer.

It goes without saying that using cocaine, heroin, methamphetamines and other drugs is dangerous for countless reasons, including their highly toxic impact on the liver.

TOXIC FOODS

Food is nature's medicine, but unfortunately, not all food should be used to fill the prescription. Whenever possible, eat organic foods, which are grown without pesticides and artificial fertilizers. If you cannot afford to buy only organic foods, try to at least select organic version of the following, which are consistently highest in pesticide contamination when grown with conventional farming practices. A general rule of thumb is to buy organic when you are going to eat the entire food, including skin.

- apples
- bell peppers
- celery
- cherries
- grapes
- nectarine
- peaches
- pears
- potatoes
- red raspberries
- spinach
- strawberries

Also avoid nitrates and nitrites used to cure food like ham, hotdogs and deli meats.

Heavy metals abound in certain foods, particularly large salt-water fish that are high on the food chain. Consume them in moderation, not more than once or twice a month.

There is another toxin that can lurk in food. Aflatoxin (*Aspergillus flavus*), a fungus that can grow on grains such as corn and rice and nuts that have not been properly stored, is a known carcinogen. Fermented foods, including milk and soy beans, can also be contaminated. When a person is exposed to such contaminated foods over a long period of time, aflatoxins can damage a gene that normally regulates excessive cell growth.

Aflatoxin is not considered a serious problem in the United States, where measures have been introduced to prevent grains in storage from developing mold and requires tests for aflatoxins. But it is a significant factor impacting the incidence of liver cancer in undeveloped countries, particularly those with warm climates where molds are more common. In Johannesburg, South Africa, for example, where cornmeal is a staple food, natives are 27 times likely to get liver cancer than individuals in the U.S.; the rate is 270 times greater in Mozambique. Hepatitis B and C are also common throughout Africa, adding to the risk.

Eating green vegetables or taking chlorophyllin supplements appears to significantly reduce the amount of aflatoxin byproducts that can damage DNA. Residents of Oidong, China, have a high rate of liver cancer, in part from eating foods contaminated with aflatoxins. Researchers from Johns Hopkins divided 180 healthy people from this part of China into two groups and had people in one group take 300 mgs of chlorophyllin daily. The other half received a placebo. After four months, analysis of blood and urine samples showed that those who took the chlorophyllin had a 55 percent reduction in aflatoxin damage to their DNA. The research suggests that the chlorophyllin blocks the absorption of aflatoxins and carcinogens.

Fatty foods put stress on the liver, especially chowing down on foods fried in rancid fats, which contain lipid peroxides that are toxic to the liver. Fast food French fries, anyone?

The jury is out on coffee. Old wisdom says that caffeine puts stress on the liver, too. But a fairly substantial body of new research praises coffee's antioxidant properties, and not just because of the caffeine.

Kaiser Permanente researchers extend the benefits of coffee to the liver and note a specific protective effect against alcoholic cirrhosis. Plus, they say, the more coffee a person consumes, the lower the risk of dying from alcoholic cirrhosis.

People drinking one cup of

Coffee crops are also highly contaminated with pesticides. If you're a coffee lover be sure to buy organic. There are increasingly documented health benefits associated with moderate coffee drinking.

coffee a day were 20 percent less likely to have alcoholic cirrhosis. People drinking two or three cups were 40 percent less likely
to have alcoholic cirrhosis. For people who drank four or more
cups of coffee a day, there was an 80 percent reduction in risk.

Researchers conclude it is not caffeine, because tea drinkers
did not receive the same liver disease protective benefit as coffee
drinkers.

My take: I don't recommend coffee as an effective remedy for
long-term liver damage that can come from too much drinking
or alcoholism. It doesn't make sense to damage your liver with
excessive drinking and then try to repair it with coffee.

Industrial Toxins

As with other forms of cancer, individuals who work in certain sectors show unusually high rates of liver cancer. In this
case, workers who are regularly exposed to heavy metals such as
mercury, lead and cadmium have higher rates of liver cancer.

And it doesn't stop there. Workers who are regularly exposed
to gasoline, diesel fuel, motor oil and degreasing chemicals, all
of which can be absorbed by inhaling fumes or through the skin,
are at higher risk. Exposure to vinyl chloride used to make
polyvinyl chloride (PVC), a form of plastic, is associated with
two rare forms of liver cancer called angiosarcoma and hemangiosarcoma that begin in the blood vessels of the liver.

Medical personnel and others exposed to radiation suffer
increased risk for liver cancer, with the disease manifesting itself
as long as 50 years after exposure. For example, a contrast dye
called Thorotrast, which once was given to patients before having an X-ray, was banned half a century ago in the U.S. after
being linked to angiosarcoma and hemangiosarcoma. The chemical continued to show its ill effects for decades afterward.

In the agricultural sector, farm workers who are exposed to
pesticides such as chlordane, lindane, 2-4-5-T and dioxin face
heightened risk of liver damage, which can result in liver cancer.

Like DDT, which was also associated with liver cancer before it was banned in this country, these toxins collect in body fat.

Even if you don't work in any of these industries, the wisest policy is to avoid or minimize exposure to any of these substances.

In addition to toxins you ingest, others from personal care and household cleaning products can enter your body through your nasal passages or skin.

Take a quick inventory of your home and get rid of anything that contains the following known carcinogens:

- parabens (found in adult and baby shampoo and many other products)

- formaldehyde (found in nail polish and numerous types of household cleaners)

- phthalates (found in all types of plastics)

- bisphenol-A (also found in plastics and food can liners)

- petroleum byproducts (found in shampoos and soaps)

- triclosan (found in antibacterial soaps)

- lead (found in lipstick and men's hair color)

- APEs (found in detergents, disposable diapers, all-purpose cleaners and laundry detergents)

- organochlorines (found in pesticides, detergents, degreasers and bleaches)

- styrene (found in plastic food wrap, insulated cups, PVC piping and carpet backing)

This is just the tip of the iceberg. There are many, many more toxic substances in our daily lives. Do a little research on your own. You'll be shocked!

The poison arsenic, which can contaminate water supplies, has also been linked to the development of liver cancer. Recent reports of high arsenic content in all types of rice, apparently extracted from the soil, are particularly worrisome. These and many other chemicals irritate the liver; if irritation is chronic, it can cause the cells to divide abnormally in their attempt to repair damage. The more the cells divide, the greater the chance that it will lead to cancer.

The importance of detoxification

It is important to understand that it is not just exposure to a vast array of environmental poisons that create waste products within the body. The normal metabolic processes of converting food into energy as well as ongoing cellular biochemical activity also regularly generate waste products. The body has a built-in defensive mechanism for detoxification, which is handled by enzymes.

In the simplest terms, there are two phases in the detoxification process. In Phase I, enzymes change the chemical structure of the toxin by adding either a single nitrogen or oxygen molecule. This process creates free radicals, which are actually more toxic than the original toxin. In Phase II, other enzymes take over, enabling antioxidants to bond with and neutralize free radicals, while also making them water-soluble, so they can easily be washed from the body. It is not hard to understand that if the body is deficient in antioxidants, the free radicals created in Phase I can inflict damage.

Some of the genes that partake in these two phases have been identified. Alterations in the DNA of these genes can impact the efficiency of the detoxification process, making them function too slowly or too quickly. To a certain extent, the foods you eat can impact the efficiency of these genes. For example, the effectiveness of Phase I enzymes can be negatively impacted by eating lots of smoked or cured meats, which contain nitrosamines. Conversely, if enzymes are too "enthusiastic" about attacking a toxin, they may create even more dangerous byproducts and the creation of more free radicals.

For this reason and because our environment is more polluted than ever, our bodies often need a helping hand to remove toxins. Understand that the liver is not alone in its role as chief detoxifier. Like a well-run military campaign, the liver's job is complemented by the work of other "battalions," in this case, the kidneys and intestines. The liver's role is to destroy or disarm toxins and then change them into a water-soluble form the kidneys can excrete in urine. The kidneys are the primary filters for disposing of water-soluble toxins. The intestines eliminate harmful waste through regular bowel movements.

Dietary deterrents

By now, it must be clear that everything you can do to detoxify your body by removing waste products and boosting your immune system is integral to protecting yourself against liver cancer.

Eating plenty of organic vegetables and a moderate amount of fruit, whole grains, legumes, nuts and seeds will provide your body with the nutrients that promote liver health. For your liver to do its life-preserving work most effectively, it needs the following nutrients:

- *Fiber* binds with bile to eliminate fat-soluble toxins. When there is not enough fiber in the diet, chronic constipation can cause the body to reabsorb toxins and cholesterol. Foods rich in fiber include vegetables, legumes and fruit.

- *Antioxidants* such as vitamins C and E and beta carotene protect and help heal damage to the liver. Good sources of vitamin C include vegetables in the cabbage family, spinach, asparagus and bell peppers as well as citrus fruits, strawberries, mangoes, papaya and kiwi fruit. vitamin E can be found in nuts and seeds, avocados, leafy green vegetables and whole grains.

- *The B vitamins* choline, betaine, vitamin B_6, folic acid, and vitamin B_{12} assist in fat metabolism. Foods that supply B complex vitamins include nutritional yeast, nuts, seeds and whole grains such as brown rice, buckwheat and wild rice (which is not actually a grain). The B vitamins methionine and cysteine (found in the cabbage family, onions and garlic, egg yolks, red peppers, sesame seeds, whole grains, and legumes) help convert fat-soluble toxins to water-soluble ones so they can be excreted in urine. All B vitamins may be depleted by excessive alcohol consumption or other toxic exposure.

- *Calcium glucarate and other trace minerals* from cruciferous vegetables like broccoli, cauliflower and cabbage that helps your body flush out hydrocarbons from gas, coal and oil exhaust fumes as well as nitrosamines, and helps lower levels of beta-glucuronidase, a dangerous enzyme that prevents detoxification in your body and instead allows pollutants to re-enter your bloodstream and damage your cells.

A proper diet also allows you to quickly replace nutrients that some detox programs may wash away along with toxins.

The cabbage family

Diet also plays an important part in Phase II of the detoxification process. In addition to calcium glucarate, cruciferous vegetables all contain glucosinolates, a type of phytochemical that activates the body's natural enzymes to excrete toxic substances. They also boost levels of glutathione that helps the liver expel toxins. In addition to the veggies mentioned above, the cruciferous vegetable family includes arugula, bok choy, broccoli, Brussels sprouts, chard, daikon radish, kale, kohlrabi, mustard greens, radishes, parsnips, turnips (and their greens) and watercress.

The maximum benefit from these vegetables results from eating them raw. Try to have at least two raw servings a week: nosh on radishes, make a salad of watercress or arugula, dip broccoli florets into hummus. When you do cook the crucifers, make sure to gently and quickly steam or stir-fry them so they retain their color and shape along with the nutrients. By all means, don't boil or otherwise overcook them, which makes them change color and release sulphides, which account for the unpleasant odor when crucifers are overcooked.

Onions and kin

Known as alliums, onions and garlic also increase the activity of enzymes that help the body excrete toxins more quickly, thanks to pungent compounds called allyl sulphides. When you cut or crush garlic, a chemical called alliin combines with the enzyme allinase to produce allicin, which has been shown to reduce the risk for cancer as well as heart disease. Onions appear to act in a similar way, although they are not as potent as garlic. Vegetables in the allium family (which include chives, leeks, scallions and shallots) also contain quercitin, which along with allicin, is an antioxidant. The allium family also has probiotic properties, enhancing intestinal flora.

Try to eat garlic and onions every day and to have about five cloves of garlic a week. Fortunately, cooking destroys only about 10 percent of garlic and onion's nutritional value, so there is no need to eat them raw if they disagree with you. On the other hand, garlic in a pesto sauce or aioli is delicious as are chopped scallions or chives over an omelet or in a salad. If you are unable to tolerate fresh garlic in any form, use an aged garlic supplement that contains allicin instead.

Additional detoxifying foods

The kidneys are also involved in detoxifying the body and often work in tandem with the liver. Any food that has a diuretic effect helps cleanse the body of toxins. Such foods include artichokes (which also protect the liver), asparagus (which also helps maintain "good" intestinal bacteria), fennel, parsley, spinach and watercress.

A few other foods worthy of special mention for their detoxifying properties include:

- Apples cleanse both the liver and kidneys and help excrete cholesterol and heavy metals.

- Beets contain a number of detoxifying important substances, including: betaine, betalains, fiber, iron, betacyanin, folate, and betanin. Pectin, a fiber found in beets, can also help flush the toxins that have been removed from the liver, carrying them out of the system instead of being reabsorbed by the body. (*Note:* Beets contain a lot of sugar and so can cause weight gain.)

- Cranberry is well known for its ability to fight bacteria in the bladder, urinary tract and kidneys, enhancing the detoxification process.

- Ginger, used in a bath or as a tea, induces sweating and help flush out toxins.

- Lemon and apple cider vinegar stimulate the release of enzymes to hasten detoxification.

The role of supplements

As I explained in the food section above, nutritional deficiencies make it difficult for your liver to do its job of removing toxins, and inadequate levels of antioxidants, in particular, can actually increase the toxic load on your body if free radicals are not promptly eliminated. As part of your insurance policy for good health and longevity, the antioxidant supplements I have discussed in other chapters are essential for liver health. There are also a few other supplements that should have starring roles in your liver-protection program.

Alpha lipoic acid

The antioxidant alpha lipoic acid (ALA) appears to have a remarkable ability to regenerate a damaged liver. In the U.S., Burton Berkson, MD, has championed its use for the last 30 years. He originally gave ALA in intravenous or oral form to people who had eaten mushrooms that contain certain toxins, which typically damage the liver irreparably and result in death. Many of Dr. Berkson's mushroom-poisoned patients have survived and their liver function returned to normal.

ALA also has the ability to chelate heavy metals, binding with them so they can be excreted. ALA has also inhibited oxidation of both copper and iron in animals.

Dr. Berkson also used ALA to treat three patients with hepatitis C who were awaiting a liver transplant. They were also given other antioxidants silymarin (milk thistle) and selenium as well as vitamins B, C and E and a mineral supplement. The patients also were given a dietary and exercise regimen and instructions to avoid stress. All three individuals were able to avoid having a liver transplant and felt healthy a year later. As a side note, a year's treatment with ALA, silymarin and selenium costs less than $2,000 while a liver transplant costs more than $300,000.

Although treatment with ALA is considered "alternative" in the U.S., Europeans have used it to treat a variety of liver ailments for many years.

Optimal daily dose: 600 mg

Vitamin K

This nutrient may not be familiar to most people, but this is a fat-soluble vitamin produced in the intestines and found in leafy green vegetables such as spinach and broccoli, grains and some meats and cheeses. It seems to be of benefit in both preventing and fighting liver cancer. Excess amounts of vitamin K are stored in the liver for future use. A recent Japanese study indicates that vitamin K is strongly associated with a reduction in risk for liver cancer among those at greatest risk, namely people with viral cirrhosis, caused by diseases such as hepatitis C. vitamin K appears to inhibit the growth of liver cancer cells. Only two of 19 women with viral hepatitis who were given 45 mgs a day of vitamin K developed liver cancer, compared to nine of 19 who received a placebo, yielding a 90 percent decrease in liver cancer.

Another Japanese study has shown that patients with liver cancer who have a vitamin K deficiency have a poorer chance of survival than those with adequate levels. Other studies have found that vitamin K slowed the progression of liver cancer.

Optimal daily dose: 100–300 mcg

Note: You must use caution if you are taking blood thinners, because vitamin K can dangerously thin your blood. Consult your health care practitioner.

CHAPTER 18

Lung Cancer

Lung cancer is the fourth most prevalent cancer in the U.S. Nonmelanoma skin cancer, prostate cancer and breast cancer respectively hold the top three places in this notorious list.

There are two main types of lung cancer: non-small cell lung cancer and small cell lung cancer. Non-small cell lung cancer is far more common (about 85 percent of those diagnosed), grows and spreads more slowly than small cell lung cancer and is treated differently.

Overall, the five-year survival rate for lung cancer is only 15 percent, although this dismal prediction jumps to 49 percent if diagnosis is made while the disease is still confined to the lungs. As always, early detection is key to an optimistic outcome.

The estimated number of new cases of lung and bronchus cancer in the U.S. in 2013 is 228,190 with an estimated 159,480 deaths.

From 2005–2009, the median age at death for cancer of the lung and bronchus was 72 years of age with over 60 percent of deaths from lung cancer in the 65- to 84-year-old age group. This is due to the fact that lung cancer can take decades to develop and often isn't diagnosed until the symptoms have greatly advanced and is likely related to smoking and sadly, even those who have quit smoking for decades.

African-American men have the highest incidence at 99.9 per
100,000 men while white women and black women have similar
rates or 55.1 and 52.6 per 100,000 women, respectively.

The smoking gun

Tobacco use is the number one cause of lung cancer but people
who don't smoke can also develop cancer. Radon is the second
greatest cause of lung cancer. I'll talk more about that in a
moment. Whether or not you smoke, it is important for you to
protect your body from smoke, which includes avoiding secondhand smoke from others.

If you do smoke, talk with an expert about quitting. It's
never too late to quit. And if you do have lung cancer, quitting
may reduce the chance of it spreading or another type of cancer developing.

In 1950, British epidemiologist Rich Doll, MD, who was later
knighted for his work, published a groundbreaking study linking
smoking to lung cancer. Doll gave up smoking two-thirds of the
way through his research as the outcome became clear, but it was a
decade before most people sat up and took notice. Instead, they
still embraced the ubiquitous television advertisements showing
white-coated "doctors" touting the stress-relieving benefits of
smoking.

In 1965, almost 42 percent of Americans over the age of
18 were smoking; by 2010, it had nearly been cut in half to
21.5 percent.

Nonetheless, the disease continues to be a major killer and is
the leading cause of cancer deaths in the U.S. The good news is
that the incidence of lung cancer has been decreasing since the
late1980s among men in North America, Australia, New
Zealand and northwestern Europe. However, the rate continues
to increase among women in these countries, and among both
men and women in southern and Eastern Europe. This fact cor-
relates with statistics showing that the decline in smoking has

It is estimated that 87 percent of lung cancer is cause by cigarette smoking. Smokers are about 20 times more likely to get lung cancer than non-smokers. The tar in tobacco includes more than 4,800 chemicals, 69 of which are known carcinogens, another 140 or more of which are likely carcinogens and 200 of which are heavy metals, which are toxic in their own right. On the short list are:

- Acetone, a poison used in nail polish remover

- Ammonia, another poison used in glass cleaners, toilet cleaners and other cleaning products

- Arsenic, a well-known poison

- Butane, used in lighter fluid

- Cadmium, a poisonous metal used in making batteries

- Nickel, a heavy metal

- Nicotine, an addictive drug and poison used as an insecticide

- Carbon monoxide, a deadly gas in car exhaust

- DDT/Dieldrin, a deadly insecticide that has been banned for more than 30 years but is still found in human tissues

- Ethanol, a form of alcohol

- Formaldehyde, a poison used by undertakers to preserve corpses

- Hexamine, a known carcinogen used in barbecue lighter fluid

- Hydrogen cyanide, a poison used in execution by injection

- Methane, sewer gas

- Methanol, rocket fuel

- Napthalene, a carcinogen and the active ingredient in mothballs

- PAHs (polycyclic aromatic hydrocarbons)

- TSNAs (tobacco-specific nitrosamines carcinogens)

- Toluene, a poison and industrial solvent

been sharper among men than women, possibly in part because smoking helps suppress appetite and women tend to have more concerns about weight control. Just as an aside, I have talked about weight control a great deal in this book, but smoking is a far greater hazard to your health. If you stop smoking and put on a few pounds, I can work with you on that. Don't wait. Stop smoking today!

Tragically, although the clear connection between smoking and lung cancer has been established for more than half a century, awareness has not resulted in universal behavior changes. A fifth of the American adult population continues to smoke; in adults with less than a high school education it remains high at 33.3 percent. And in high school students, smoking has increased to 35 percent.

Increases in smoking continue at alarming rates among women and people in certain other parts of the world. Lung cancer has been the most common cancer in the world for several decades, and by 2008, there were an estimated 1.61 million new cases, representing 12.7 percent of all new cancer diagnoses. It was also the most common cause of death from cancer, with 1.38 million deaths (18.2 percent of the total cancer deaths) worldwide. The majority of the cases now occur in the developing countries (55 percent).

Lung cancer is still the most common cancer in men worldwide (1.1 million cases, 16.5 percent of the total), with high rates in central-eastern and southern Europe, North America and Eastern Asia. In women, incidence rates are generally lower, but, worldwide, lung cancer is now the fourth most frequent cancer of women (516,000 cases, 8.5 percent of all cancers) and the second most common cause of death from cancer (427,000 deaths, 12.8 percent of the total). The highest incidence rate is observed in North America (where lung cancer it is now the second most frequent cancer in women), and the lowest in Middle Africa (15th most frequent cancer).

Assessing your risk

Habit, addiction, ignorance and the mistaken belief that "it won't happen to me" mean that lung cancer will surely continue to strike millions of people. And the more and the longer a person smokes, the greater his or her risk. A recent study found that people who smoked two or more packs of cigarettes a day are 20 times more likely to get lung cancer than non-smokers.

Cigar and pipe smoking are considered almost as dangerous as cigarette smoking in causing lung cancer. Nor do low-tar cigarettes appear to significantly reduce the risk; they reduce the tar and nicotine yields from an average of 37 and 2.7 mg to 12 and 0.85 mg.

The only way for smokers to really cut their risk is to stop smoking as soon as possible! Fortunately, the longer an ex-smoker stays "clean," the more his or her risk for lung cancer decreases, although it can take 10 to 15 years before an ex-smoker's risk is comparable to that of people who have never smoked.

If you have already had lung cancer, you are at elevated risk for developing it again. Having a parent or sibling who has had the diseases appears to slightly increase risk. Many studies are pointing to possible genetic components in developing lung cancer. Certain respiratory diseases, such as tuberculosis and beryllioisis or silicosis (both caused by inhaling certain minerals), can damage and scar the lungs, also increasing one's risk.

People who have been irradiated in the chest area for cancer are at higher risk for lung cancer, and the risk escalates if they also smoke. However, women who were irradiated after breast cancer surgery, but do not smoke, are not at increased risk for lung cancer.

What about pot?

Is smoking marijuana also risky business? Pot does have more tar than tobacco and it does contain many of the same cancer-causing substances found in tobacco. Typically, smokers inhale marijuana deeply and hold the smoke in the lungs for a long time. But studies have not linked marijuana use to lung cancer (although current research does suggest an association between marijuana smoking and mouth and throat cancers).

Secondhand smoke

Even people who have never taken so much as a puff of tobacco can develop lung cancer. Secondhand smoke, also known as environmental tobacco smoke (ETS), may be the culprit in many cases. It is estimated that ETS is to blame for almost a third of all lung cancer cases. While the common assumption that secondhand smoke is less dangerous than that inhaled by smokers, the particles are actually smaller than those in "primary" tobacco smoke, meaning they are more easily inhaled and thus more apt to accumulate in the lungs.

Worldwide in 2004, 40 percent of children, 33 percent of male non-smokers and 35 percent of female non-smokers were exposed to secondhand smoke. This exposure was estimated to have caused 603,000 deaths, with 21,400 of these from lung cancer (as well as 379,000 deaths from heart disease, 165,000 from lower respiratory infections and 36,900 from asthma).

Growing up in a household in which adults smoke—as 20 percent of children do—particularly increases risk. Non-smoking husbands and wives of smokers have a 30 percent greater risk of developing lung cancer than those married to non-smokers. Likewise, people who are exposed to second hand tobacco smoke in the workplace are also at heightened risk.

A report issued by the Surgeon General in June of 2006 stressed that no amount of secondhand smoke is safe, meaning smoke-free spaces, as opposed to areas set aside within one space, are essential. Based upon current research, the report also cites the exposure to secondhand smoke as responsible for a 20 to 30 percent increased risk for lung cancer, as well as a 25 to 30

percent increased risk for heart disease. About 430 infants suc-
cumbed to sudden infant death syndrome (SIDS) in 2005 alone
as a result of secondhand smoke. Respiratory problems, ear
infections and asthma attacks are other consequences children
may experience, thanks to adults lighting up in the home.

The toxic environment

On the most basic level, the job of your lungs is to add oxygen
to your blood with each inhaled breath and to remove carbon
dioxide with every exhalation. Although the lungs are adept at
filtering out impurities, if you put a heavy burden on them, they
are almost certain to become overloaded. That is what happens
not only from smoking, but also from assaults by general air pollution and exposure to gases like radon, materials like asbestos,
heavy metals and a host of manmade chemicals like PAHs (polyaromatic hydrocarbons).

Radon

Radon gas is the runner up after tobacco smoke as the major
cause of lung cancer. This radioactive gas is a byproduct of the
natural breakdown of uranium and rises from the soil, infiltrat-
ing houses and other buildings through cracks in foundations
and walls and openings around pipes, even through well water.
Levels of radon in the soil vary geographically. Most are not high
enough to be dangerous, but because radon is odorless, tasteless
and invisible, you don't know if you have a radon problem
unless you test for it. It is estimated that one in 15 homes has a
level that could cause concern. Inexpensive test kits are available
at most hardware stores. Radon mitigation involves simple ven-
tilation systems that usually cost $1,000 or less. Miners are at
particular risk for the effects of radon gas.

Asbestos

Asbestos is a naturally occurring mineral fiber that used to be heavily utilized in construction, appearing in siding and shingles, floor tiles, textured paints, insulation, fire retardants and thousands of other products. Several asbestos products have been banned and most builders prefer not to use products that contain it because of the health risks.

Asbestos is generally found in older houses; if it remains intact, it is not considered a health hazard. It becomes dangerous when insulation, for example, degrades or when remodeling work disturbs or dislodges asbestos-based products, releasing minute fibers into the air. Too small to see, these fibers can embed themselves in the lungs and respiratory tract and damage cells. Removal and disposal of asbestos-containing materials requires the assistance of hazardous materials experts.

Asbestos exposure is a risk factor for lung disease. Workers, such as remodeling contractors who regularly encounter asbestos, have three to four times the usual risk for lung cancer; such workers who also smoke have an eight-fold risk compared to that of other smokers. Asbestos is a culprit in causing other crippling lung diseases. Spouses and children of those exposed to asbestos in the workplace can also be exposed to asbestos by clothes brought home from a work site.

Arsenic

Exposure to this poisonous heavy metal has been demonstrated to raise the risk of developing lung cancer along with cancers of the skin, bladder, kidney and liver. It is found not only in mines and smelting plants where it is processed, but also in plants where wood preservatives, glass and pesticides are made, as well as in the products themselves. Less commonly known is that water supplies can be tainted with arsenic.

Industrial toxins

Working in industries that produce known and suspected carcinogens and other chemicals clearly puts an individual at heightened risk for many forms of cancer. Numerous studies have linked certain industries to elevated risks of lung cancer in its workers. These include workers exposed to silica dust or fiberglass; heavy metals such as beryllium, chromium, cadmium and nickel; chemicals such as benzene, vinyl chloride and nickel chromates, coal products, uranium, mustard gas and chloromethyl ethers. Working in certain industries such as smelting, mining, electroplating, welding, the manufacture of pesticides, paint, solvents batteries, ceramics or glass and nuclear energy are all at heightened risks. And when an individual who is exposed to these toxins also smokes, the risks mount still higher.

Of course, these pollutants are around all of us. As an obvious example, every time we pump gas into our cars, we are exposed to a carcinogen linked to lung cancer.

Indoor air pollution

When we think about air pollution, images of smokestacks spewing out industrial fumes come to mind. But according to the U.S. Environmental Protection Agency (EPA) our homes and offices typically contain two to five times more pollutants than the air outside, partly due to "improved" construction methods that save energy by being more airtight. Indoor air can be contaminated with cooking oils and carbon monoxide and nitrogen dioxide from unvented or improperly operating gas appliances. Exhaust from cars and trucks may leak in from the garage and street. Add to that volatile organic compounds (VOCs) off-gassing from construction materials, paints and other finishes, furnishings, dozens of cleaning supplies filled with hundreds of chemicals, and even permanent-press fabrics and fragrances in air fresheners and personal care products, to name just a few.

Almost every time we go to the supermarket, we come home with toxins in the form of bleach, drain cleaners, oven cleaners and toilet bowl cleansers, all of which are particularly irritating to the lungs as well as your eyes, nose and throat. Individuals with asthma or lung problems should never use chlorine bleach and ammonia, for example, which produce noxious fumes. Combinations of cleaning products can form lung-damaging gases. When chlorine meets ammonia or ammonia meets lye (as in some oven cleaners), chloramine gases are produced. And when chlorine meets the acids in toilet bowl cleaners, equally toxic chlorine gas is released.

Electromagnetic fields

Electromagnetic fields, like those found in electrical power lines, common household appliances like televisions, electronic devices like computers, tablets and readers and mobile phones have been weakly linked to an increased risk of certain types of cancer, including lung cancer. There is no definitive research available yet, but precautions are worthwhile if you live near high voltage power lines. You can also help neutralize the risks by unplugging electronic devices and keeping cell phones and other electronics away from you in the bedroom.

My objective is not to overwhelm you with this information but to stimulate you to change the things you can change in your environment, starting with:

- avoid secondhand smoke

- modify certain buying habits

- take proper precautions when working with certain products

- eliminate what you can

- minimize what cannot be eliminated

- don't obsess about what you might have done differently in the past

- air out your house regularly

- sleep with a window slightly open

- install a range hood that vents outdoors and see that it is properly maintained

As you will learn in the sections that follow, you can also fortify your immune system with foods and nutritional supplements that can undo some damage and prevent additional damage to your lungs.

Dietary deterrents

As I have advised in earlier chapters, your anti-lung-cancer diet will consist of plenty of (and a variety of) vegetables and some fruits for their antioxidant and anticarcinogenic benefits. Most studies suggest that the more vegetables and fruits in the diet, the less the likelihood of developing lung cancer. Several nutrients, including flavonoids, which are found in most vegetables and fruits, are likely to confer protection; a specific flavonoid found in onions and apples has been shown to be of particular value.

People who regularly eat good sources of the antioxidant beta-carotene (found in yellow and orange vegetables such as squash, sweet peppers, carrots, yams and fruits such as peaches, nectarines, oranges and grapefruits) are at lower risk for lung cancer.

Lycopene leucopenia, found in tomatoes, is well known for its protective value against prostate cancer, and it appears to confer protection against lung cancer.

I also advise the consumption of dark leafy greens, garlic, broccoli, Brussels sprouts, kale, cabbage and cauliflower, as well as berries for their anti-carcinogenic properties.

Smokers who drink green tea have decreased oxidative DNA damage, a genetic change that predisposes to cancers, including lung cancer.

Diets high in fruit are associated with a lower risk of lung cancer, and in fact, the National Cancer Institute has estimated that foods high in flavonoids, such as apples, can lower the risk of lung cancer by 50 percent.

In women, the intake of dairy products and vegetables has

been linked with a lower risk of lung cancer in smokers, and black tea with a lower risk in non-smokers.

Also valuable for both their antioxidant and anti-inflammatory benefits are fatty cold-water fish like salmon and tuna as well as nuts and seeds, which all contain valuable omega-3 fatty acids.

As lovers of sushi and sashimi know, fish is a key part of the traditional Japanese diet. Although lung cancer is less common in Japan than it is in the U.S., it is still Japan's leading cause of cancer deaths. A Japanese study completed in 2001 looked at diet to ascertain if it played a role in the development of the disease. More than 1,000 men and women who had been diagnosed with lung cancer and more than 4,000 men and women without the disease were surveyed. The researchers found that both men and women who ate cooked or raw fish five times a week or more had half the incidence of lung cancer compared to participants who ate cooked or raw fish less than once a week. On the other hand, eating dried or salted fish did not confer any benefit, which researchers speculated was a result of processing, which destroys the omega-3 fatty acids. Avoid large fish, which contain more mercury.

This same study found that women who ate tofu five or more times a week had half the risk of developing lung cancer than women who ate it less than once a week. A different study showed that higher intake of soy foods significantly reduced risk of lung cancer among lifetime nonsmokers, but not among smokers.

As always, avoid any refined foods, sugar and white flour. Eating lots of sugar or sugary foods increases risk for several cancers, including lung cancer.

When food is fried in oil at extremely high temperatures, it forms polycyclic aromatic hydrocarbons (PAH), which are also found in tobacco smoke and exhaust fumes from gasoline or diesel fuel. The harmful particles of PAH, which can cause cancer, are released into the air. A study by researchers in Singapore

Certain cooking methods are crucial to minimize your risk for lung cancer.

- Avoid any charred or blackened food that contains carcinogens.

- Minimize use of the barbecue, or precook foods to minimize their time over a hot flame.

- Avoid oil-based marinades that cause flames to flare and burn food.

- For the same reason, trim excess fat before grilling meat.

- Rely on methods that cook meat gently, such as roasting or braising.

- Sauté or stir-fry rather than deep-frying, and when doing so, use olive oil, coconut oil or grapeseed oil (which has a high flash point) instead of other oils.

found that of all cooking oils, vegetable oil is the most dangerous, although corn and olive oil also pose a risk.

Deep-frying French fries produced particularly large amounts of PAHs. The researchers also found that deep-frying, which is typical in many parts of Asia, released more PAHs into the air than the stir-frying, which characterizes Chinese cuisine. Indian food is typically simmered or boiled, which minimizes hydrocarbons. Repeated exposure to these hydrocarbons increases the chance of developing lung as well as breast and bladder cancer.

The role of supplements

If this chapter seems like a real downer, I actually feel tremendously optimistic about the fact that although up to 90 percent of lung cancer in the U.S. is attributed to cigarette smoking, only

10 to 20 percent of smokers actually develop lung cancer. This means that despite tobacco's assault on their lungs, the vast majority of our bodies are able to defend us from this deadly disease. What is it about diet, supplement regimens and lifestyles that protect some people?

I am convinced that it is a matter of a healthy immune system, which is linked to diet and supplement intake, as well as genetic strengths or predispositions. My advice is to supplement a healthy low-carbohydrate diet with a mix of antioxidants, anti-inflammatory and anticarcinogenic nutrients in supplement form.

Diet and supplements may not be enough to stave off all disease, but research continues to confirm the benefits of nutrition on numerous forms of cancer. Some of these findings are offered here. *All* of the research, however, states very clearly that *not* smoking is the most successful means of avoiding lung cancer, and some of them showed that taking supplements to combat lung cancer was more effective when the patient quit smoking.

Note that there is more general information on many of these supplements in Chapter 1 and in the opening section on cancer. In addition, try this:

Whey protein

Whey protein is a mixture of globular proteins isolated from whey, the liquid material created as a by-product of cheese production. High heat (such as the sustained high temperatures above 72° C associated with the pasteurization process) denatures whey proteins.

Undenatured whey protein appears to raise levels of glutathione, known as the body's master antioxidant, which allows the liver to better perform its detoxifying activities.

It appears that cancer cells have higher levels of glutathione than normal cells, making them stronger and more difficult to kill than healthy cells. Lung cancer cells actually have levels seven times higher than normal lung cells. Consuming whey protein raises the level of glutathione in normal cells, making them stronger. Whey does the same to malignant cells, but in this case, after the level of glutathione rises, it "peaks out" and then drops, causing the cancer cells to weaken and ultimately shut off. This may be why Japanese studies on rats have found that feeding them bovine lactoferrin (bLF), a component of whey protein, inhibited development of lung cancer (as well as colon, esophagus and bladder cancers).

Optimal daily dose: 20 grams

In Summary

- Avoid lung cancer by not smoking. If you do smoke, stop NOW, whatever it takes.

- As with any cancer, early detection is the key to defeating this disease.

- Avoid secondhand smoke as well as any indoor or outdoor air pollutants possible.

- Check your home for toxic radon levels and do what you need to do to bring those levels to safe ranges and limit your exposure to other chemicals that are toxic to your lungs.

- The more vegetables and fruits in your diet, the less the likelihood you have of developing lung cancer. Adding certain supplements also seems to help protect against lung cancer.

CHAPTER 19

Colorectal Cancer

One of the few bright spots in the dismal terrain of cancer is that of colon cancer, more properly called colorectal cancer. Since 1991, death rates from colon cancer have decreased by more than 30 percent. This is due in large part to screening processes that find polyps, which can be removed before they turn into tumors, and enable diagnosis while the disease is still in its early stages.

Nonetheless, with the exception of nonmelanoma skin cancers, colorectal cancer is the third most common form of cancer in the U.S. In 2013, the American Cancer Society estimates that more than 102,000 new cases of colon cancer will be diagnosed as well as more than 40,000 new cases of rectal cancer. About 50,000 people will die from the two diseases.

Before we go any further, here is a short anatomy lesson on territory with which many of us are not familiar. The colon comprises most of the large intestine, which runs up one side of your abdomen, across the top and down the other side for about six feet, where it meets the rectum, which in turn gives way to the six-inch-long anal canal, ending in the anus.

The first step in preventing colorectal cancer is to detect a precancerous condition with regular tests. The simplest test, which the American Cancer Society suggests be performed once a year after age 50 for those with average risk, is known as the fecal occult blood test (FOBT), which reveals hidden blood in the stool. You obtain a kit and provide a stool sample in the privacy of your home. Then you give this to your physician who sends it to a laboratory for analysis.

After a lab analysis, if blood is present, you will be advised to have further tests to determine the source of the bleeding. If necessary, your doctor will schedule you for a colonoscopy, in which the entire colon is scanned and, if necessary, any polyps are removed. A colonoscopy requires mild sedation for comfort. Even with no blood in the stool, people with average risk factors should have either a sigmoidoscopy or a colonoscopy at age 50 and every 10 years.

Virtual colonoscopies, new low-radiation noninvasive screenings, are becoming increasingly popular and should be repeated every five years.

If you have a family history of colorectal cancer or other heightened risk factors, your physician may suggest you start screening before age 50 and with greater frequency.

Assessing your risk

The usual suspects

Like most other forms of cancer, your risk for colorectal cancer increases with age. People aged 50 or older are far more susceptible. Likewise, inactivity increases your risk. Not surprisingly, being significantly overweight (especially around the waist, which is often a sign of impaired ability to metabolize insulin, and especially for men) stacks the deck against you.

However, the association between obesity and colorectal cancer is weaker for women than it is for men. One possible explanation is that estrogen appears to be protective in the case of colon cancer, in contrast to its role in breast, uterine and ovarian cancers.

One study did find an increased risk of colon cancer among women who carried their weight in their middle *and* were inactive.

It would appear that being physically active can override the effects of the spare tire of fat. Waistline obesity is also associated with a predisposition to blood sugar and insulin imbalances and the development of diabetes, so it should come as no surprise that having diabetes or high insulin levels appears to be another risk factor for colorectal cancer.

The tobacco connection

As with other forms of cancer, smoking heightens risk for colorectal cancer. According to a major cancer prevention study, which began in 1982 and followed almost 800,000 individuals for 14 years, smokers had a 30 to 40 percent greater chance of dying from colorectal cancer than nonsmokers.

The alcohol connection

Joe Six Pack won't like to hear this, but there is undeniable evidence that drinking beer is associated with precancerous changes in the colon as well as with both rectal and colon cancer. Don't think that switching to Scotch or other spirits gets you out of the woods. Alcohol can indirectly damage DNA, leading to cancer, and some studies have found that drinking any kind of alcohol is associated with colorectal cancers.

On the other hand, if you drink, you might want to consider switching to wine in moderation, of course. It appears that red wine (and perhaps white as well) protects not just the heart but the colon as well if your drinking is moderate: one drink a day for women and two for men. The preventative effects of wine may be due to the presence of resveratrol, an antioxidant and antibiotic in the skins of grapes, which has the ability to interfere with the growth and spread of cancer cells.

Disease history

If you've had colon or rectal cancer, it is more likely to reappear than in someone who has never had the disease. A family history of colon or rectal cancer plays a role in the risk game.

A NEW CULPRIT: INFLAMMATION

Inflammation is the body's normal response to injury or infection. However, inflammation can spiral out of control.

The relationship of inflammation and colon cancer is a complex one. People who already have inflammation in the gastrointestinal (GI) tract in the form of irritable bowel syndrome, inflammatory bowel diseases like ulcerative colitis or Crohn's disease are at heightened risk of developing colorectal cancer.

Higher levels of an enzyme called prostaglandin E-2 have been found in the colons of people with colorectal cancer, indicating inflammation was present in the colon. Prostaglandins help control inflammation, but some prostaglandins, including E-2, can overcorrect and actually become inflammatory agents themselves.

Inhibiting this enzyme with a variety of anti-inflammatory agents can shrink tumors and keep them from developing in the first place. Aspirin and other NSAIDs (nonsteroidal anti-inflammatory drugs), fish oils and vegetables and fruits all lower prostaglandin levels and reduce inflammation. Regular use of aspirin by individuals at risk for colon cancer has been shown to significantly reduce the incidence of cancer, perhaps because it acts as a COX inhibitor, preventing the production of prostaglandin-2. But too much aspirin can cause serious GI bleeds and even death.

Being at a healthy body weight and engaging in regular exercise also reduces inflammation.

Diet plays a large role in causing or suppressing inflammation, which is provoked by foods with an acid pH. It's especially helpful to load up on alkaline vegetables and fruits, including dark green vegetables (spinach, endive, kale, cucumber, broccoli, celery and avocado), orange vegetables (sweet potato, carrot, acorn or butternut squash and pumpkin), root vegetables (radish, turnip, beet and parsnip), some legumes (lima, white navy, soy and green beans and tofu), and asparagus, onions, garlic, okra, artichoke and zucchini.

The closer your relatives and the younger they were when they became ill, the higher your risk.

A number of other diseases and conditions are also cause to stay on high alert. Women who have or have had ovarian, uterine (endometrial) or breast cancer have higher than usual odds of developing colorectal cancer. A history of colon polyps is another added risk, as is having had ulcerative colitis or Crohn's disease for 10 or more years.

Finally genetic mutations can play a role, and they are more common in certain ethnic groups, including Ashkenazi Jews. They predispose individuals to certain hereditary forms of colon cancer, including familial adenomatous polyposis (FAP) and hereditary nonpolyposis colon cancer (HNPCC), also known as Lynch Syndrome. People with these genes are at extraordinarily high risk of colorectal cancer. You can be tested for the mutated gene that can cause FAP or HNPCC, and if you have it, you need to undergo more frequent testing to treat the disease at as early as possible.

Dietary deterrents

Research suggests that up to 35 percent of cancers are related to poor diet and it is not surprising that if you spend your life eating junk, it will show in your digestive tract in the long term, particularly on the last leg of its journey through your body.

Fruits and vegetables

The familiar refrain of "eat your veggies" is particularly apt in the case of colorectal cancer prevention, not just for the multiple nutrients they contain but also for their fiber, which helps move food and waste through your digestive tract and promotes regularity. Individuals who eat a greater variety of vegetables have a dramatically lower risk of colorectal cancer. I recommend you eat at least seven servings (and preferably more) of low-carbohydrate vegetables a day and at least one serving of low-carb berries or other fruit.

Researchers have looked at the effect of eating various vegetable and fruit groups in populations over time to determine their role in reducing the risk of colon cancer. Vegetables and fruits are known to be rich sources of a variety of cancer preventive nutrients. For example, the antioxidants called

One serving is equal to:
$1/2$ cup broccoli
2 cups lettuce
$1/2$ cup green beans
$1/2$ cup mushrooms
$1/2$ cup berries

carotenoids found in many vegetables and fruits are recognized as protective against many forms of cancer. Lutein, a specific carotenoid found in spinach, lettuce and other leafy greens, broccoli, tomatoes, carrots, celery and oranges (as well as eggs), appears to be particularly effective in reducing the risk of particular types and stages of colon cancer.

Cruciferous vegetables (*Brassicae*) are also associated with a reduced risk for colorectal cancers. They include kale, collards, Chinese broccoli (gai laan), cabbage, Brussels sprouts, kohlrabi, numerous types of broccoli, cauliflower, bok choy, mizuna, flowering cabbage, Chinese/napa cabbage, turnip, rutabaga, canola/ rapeseed, mustard seeds, tatsoi, radish, daikon, horseradish, wasabi, arugula, watercress and cress.

The red meat question

Many people believe that the consumption of red meat with its saturated fat is an increased risk factor for cancer. Certainly, a number of studies have concluded that meat *per se* is a culprit.

But I beg to differ, both from my clinical observations and because there are several huge flaws in the structure of all of these studies.

As a practitioner who worked at the side of the pioneering Dr. Robert C. Atkins and who prescribes a low-carbohydrate, low-glycemic dietary approach for most of my patients (please refer to my *Fight Fat with Fat Diet* book and website), my experience is completely at odds with this assumption.

Many of Dr. Atkins' patients, some who had been with him for up to 20 years, are now my patients. This means that I have medical records for people who have been eating a high-protein diet for up to 30 years. Only a fraction of them have developed cancer in any form.

When it comes to the research, there are at least four reasons why studies on meat consumption are flawed.

1. The meat that 99.9 percent of the population eats is not organic, meaning the animals were pumped full of hormones to increase their weight, given prophylactic antibiotics to prevent disease in cramped conditions and fed grain treated with hormone-disrupting pesticides. Unless studies looked at the effect over years of conventionally farmed meat compared to organic meat, there is no way to ascertain what effect, if any, was the meat itself or the hormones, antibiotics or pesticides, either in combination or as individual factors.

2. The studies did not distinguish between people who ate both red meat and "bad" carbohydrates such as baked goods made with flour, sugary junk foods and those who ate meat and only "good" carbohydrates like vegetables and whole grains. So how can the research conclude that the saturated fat in meat is the villain when its dietary partner ("bad carbs") is a villain that I consider far more dangerous and even deadlier when the two team up?

3. More of the fat in red meat is monounsaturated or polyunsaturated than saturated.

4. Finally, these studies do not distinguish between those who eat their hamburgers and lamb chops medium rare and those who prefer them well done. Charred meat is a known carcinogen.

That being said, I advocate a low-carbohydrate approach that includes many forms of protein. There is nothing intrinsically wrong with organically-raised beef and other red meat, but if you eat steak to the exclusion of pork, poultry, fish, eggs, cheese and soy products, you're missing out on the health benefits of other forms of protein. I also advise you to balance your fats by accompanying meat with vegetables dressed with olive oil.

Without question, you should also steer clear of meat or fish that has been processed with nitrites (which react with amino acids in the body to form cancer-causing nitrosamines), smoke or salt. This includes bacon, hot dogs, salami and most other cold cuts as well as cured hams, all of which have been particularly linked to the development of colon cancer. Citizens of Germany, Austria, Poland and the Czech Republic, where rates of colorectal cancer are high, consume a lot of their red meat in the form of sausages and other cured meats.

And the fat issue

There is also a major flaw in the theory that a low-fat diet is protective against cancer, and colorectal cancer in particular. It is important to understand that there are a number of different fats.

Some, like trans fats (also known as hydrogenated or partially hydrogenated oils) that clog your arteries and have been associated with cancer, are to be avoided at all costs.

Others, like the omega-6 fatty acids found in most vegetable oils, are to be consumed in moderation. Then there are the omega-3 fatty acids that are just plain good for you.

I consider olive oil, which is an omega-9 fatty acid, as the prince among oils for numerous reasons. In countries such as Greece, where olive oil is a staple of the diet and consumed in large quantities, the incidence of colorectal cancer is lower than other northern European countries.

How does olive oil work its wonders? According to a review of studies from 28 countries by a team at Oxford University, virgin olive oil appears to decrease the amount of deoxycyclic acid, a bile acid that promotes the progression of benign polyps to malignant colorectal tumors in the colon. By consuming olive oil, you protect your bowel by reducing the amount of deoxycyclic acid and minimizing the likelihood that cancerous cells will develop. Be sure it is the cold-pressed extra virgin type, which is rich in antioxidants, including flavonoids and lignans that also protect your cells from the normal wear and tear that comes with aging. Lignans are considered particularly good at defending against this disease. Butter, another healthy fat, also contains a powerful anticancer nutrient called butyric acid that specifically stops the growth of colon cancer cells and re-establishes a healthy lining in the large and small intestines.

The fiber question

In medical circles, the long-held belief has been that dietary fiber confers protection against colorectal cancer, perhaps by helping speed the passage of wastes through the digestive tract.

Perhaps the amount of fiber some people consumed was insufficient to prevent colorectal cancer. Perhaps other dietary components, such as fat, interact with fiber in ways not yet understood.

Nonetheless, a 2005 analysis of the recent research that examined the relationship of dietary fiber and colorectal cancer concluded that dietary fiber had a protective effect against colorectal cancer. Both men and women who consumed more dietary fiber had a lower risk of developing colorectal cancer compared to individuals who consumed little dietary fiber.

To get your daily fiber fix, eat a full complement of low-glycemic vegetables. If you are at a healthy weight, you can also enjoy whole grains, such as brown rice, oatmeal and buckwheat, and breads made from 100 percent whole grains, all in moderation. I caution you about the fat accumulation that is associated with the consumption of gluten products for many people. If you have a little belly, avoid all wheat products. Additionally (and certainly if you are limiting your intake of grains to lose weight) you should also be supplementing with B complex vitamins.

Garlic

There has been considerable research on whether eating a lot of garlic is associated with a lower risk of developing colorectal cancer. Organosulfur compounds formed when garlic is cut or crushed are associated with disease prevention and treatment. A meta-analysis of six studies found that people who ate the most garlic were about 30 percent less likely to get colorectal cancer than those who ate the least. One form of garlic apparently even has the ability to suppress the growth and progression of polyps that have already formed in the colon and rectum, effectively halting the possible progression toward cancer.

In a recent Japanese study, 37 patients who were found to have colorectal polyps as a result of a colonoscopy were divided into two groups. Some were treated with a large dose of aged garlic extract (AGE); the others were treated with a very low dose. Neither patients nor researchers knew who was getting what dose. Before starting the AGE therapy, all polyps over a certain size were removed and any small remaining polyps were measured. After six and 12 months, colonoscopies were repeated. At a year, those individuals who had a very low dose of AGE had developed more polyps, but in the high-dose group both the size and the number of polyps were significantly reduced.

Environmental hazards

Australia, Canada, the Czech Republic and Austria have an even higher incidence of colorectal cancer than the U.S. When you group these countries together with the U.S., the incidence of colorectal cancer is anywhere from three to eight times greater than in countries such as China, Colombia, Greece and India. The Japanese used to have a very low risk for the disease, but as they and other countries increasingly abandon their traditional diets and move toward a Western-type diet, rates are on the rise. As with other forms of cancer, when people from these countries emigrate to the U.S. or other high-risk countries, their risk increases but never equals that of individuals born in that country. However, second generation individuals experience about the same risk as the general population. How much of this effect is the result of diet and how much because of other environmental factors, such as toxins in the workplace, is difficult to determine.

There is presently no definitive connection between specific toxins and colorectal cancer, but there is clear evidence that deaths from colorectal cancer in the U.S. have been largely concentrated in regions that in recent history were the most industrialized, namely Massachusetts, New York, New Jersey, the North Atlantic coast and the urban centers around the Great Lakes. This supports the conclusion that manufacturing processes involving chemicals and disposal of byproducts of manufacturing processes are implicated in colorectal cancer.

Supplementing your diet

Folic Acid

Although a deficiency of folic acid is involved in many forms of cancer, its association with colorectal cancer is particularly strong. At least 20 population studies suggest that individuals with the highest folate intake are roughly 40 percent less likely to develop colorectal cancer than those with the lowest intake. Women who took a multi-vitamin that contained at least 400 micrograms of folate for 15 years or more were 75 percent less likely to develop colorectal disease than women who did not take the supplement. And not surprisingly, low intake of folate, particularly accompanied by high consumption of alcohol, increases the risk.

Research on rats shows that one of the reasons that this B vitamin may be protective against colorectal cancer is that it plays an important role in synthesizing and repairing strands of DNA. This could help explain why folate deficiency promotes—and supplementing with folate can suppress—the development of colon cancer. Colon cells regenerate and turn over quickly as opposed to liver cells or heart cells, so the potential for cancer can be multiplied if colon cells become defective.

Folic acid offers promise as a possible treatment to deter the recurrence of cancerous polyps. In one study patients who had had cancerous polyps removed and then received 1 mg of folate daily had a recurrence rate that was half that of patients who received a placebo instead.

Optimal daily dose: 400 mcg

Calcium

Numerous large studies that have followed populations over time support the association between consumption of calcium and reduced risk for colorectal cancer.

In one study, researchers compared the intake of calcium in both dietary and supplemental form by almost 4,000 individuals who had had polyps in the lower colon revealed by sigmoidoscopy compared to almost 35,000 individuals who were polyp free. In this case, the findings indicated that individuals who consumed the most calcium received the most positive effects.

Optimal daily dose: 500–1,000 mg taken with at least 250–500 mg of magnesium for mineral balance.

Vitamin D

As I mentioned in Section 1, our bodies produce vitamin D mainly through exposure of skin to sunlight. While a few foods give us minimal amounts of vitamin D, the sun is our major source. Almost all of us are vitamin D deficient, especially in winter when we're less likely to expose our skin to sunlight. The medical profession has persuaded us to protect our skin from

sunlight because of the fear of skin cancers, when actually vitamin D in the appropriate amounts is preventive for many types
of cancer, including colorectal cancer.

A number of studies have shown benefits in reducing colorectal
cancer risk when vitamin D is combined with calcium, vitamin E,
selenium and other nutrients. But vitamin D appears to have protective effects independent of other nutrients, including calcium.

One review study looked at earlier studies of vitamin D and
colon cancer conducted between 1966 and 2004, some of which
measured dietary and supplement intake and others (which could
come also from sunlight) measured blood levels. Ten of 18 studies found that individuals who did not get adequate vitamin D
had a higher risk of developing colon cancer. The authors suggested that daily intake of 1,000 IU of vitamin D cut colon cancer risk by about 50 percent.

Good dietary sources of vitamin D include oily fish such as
salmon and sardines as well as fortified milk and dairy products,
eggs and mushrooms. Other foods like orange juice and yogurt
are often fortified as well, but it can still be hard to get enough
without taking supplements.

Optimal daily dose: 3,000 IU

Fish oil

I know I've mentioned fish oil as a basic preventive for virtually every health condition, but I want to underscore its importance in terms of colorectal cancer.

A review of laboratory, animal and population-based studies
points strongly toward the advisability of consuming a diet high
in omega-3 fatty acids as a deterrent to colorectal cancer. For
example, consuming as little as 2.5 grams of fish oils daily
has been found effective in preventing the progression from
benign polyps to colon cancer. In the U.S. and other westernized
countries, the typical diet includes a ratio of polyunsaturated
fats in omega-6s to omega-3s of 20:1. The ideal for good health
and disease prevention is actually 2:1. Some omega-6 fatty acids

are highly inflammatory. The harmful ones are most frequently found in vegetable oils (especially canola oil), durum wheat, cereals and baked goods and margarine. Target the healthy omega-6s like avocados, nuts, eggs, flaxseed and poultry.

Like aspirin and other NSAIDs, fish oil works as an anti-inflammatory, which may mean that part of its effectiveness against the development of colorectal cancer is that it blocks the development of prostaglandins that can inflame the colon and lay the foundation for cancer at a later date.

Optimal daily dose: 2,000 mg/day

Turmeric

Again turmeric and its derivative, curcumin, are general cancer preventives, but it is especially helpful against colorectal cancer.

In India, where turmeric is an essential ingredient in native cuisine, there are extremely low rates of colorectal cancer. There and in many other Asian countries, turmeric is used to treat gastrointestinal disorders. Laboratory and animal studies suggest that turmeric prevents the development of colorectal cancer as well as reducing the growth of colorectal tumors.

Curcumin, an active ingredient in turmeric, is effective in suppressing the growth of cancer cells and encouraging malignant cells to die (apoptosis). It also acts as a COX-2 inhibitor, checking production of cancer-causing inflammatory prostaglandins found in bile and stomach acids.

Optimal daily dose: 1,000 mg

Green Tea Extract

I'm also reinforcing the importance of green tea and its general health benefits as well as specifically against colorectal cancer. Green tea has many cancer-protective mechanisms, including antioxidant properties, the ability to arrest the division of mutant cells, and the ability to cause cells to die at the proper time rather than reproducing wildly and indefinitely.

Several studies, mostly done in Asia, where green tea is much more commonly consumed than in the West, show a correlation between increased consumption of the beverage and reduction in the risk for colorectal cancer. The more green tea individuals drink, the less their likelihood of getting colon cancer.

A study at the Linus Pauling Institute at the Oregon State University, which has been in the forefront of green tea research, provided provocative results that could point to disease prevention for humans. The researchers used laboratory mice that are genetically predisposed to cancers of the intestinal tract. The study demonstrated that green and minimally-processed white teas are as effective as the prescription NSAID Sulindac, commonly used to prevent certain colon cancers. (Sulindac typically reduces tumor formation by about 50 percent.) One group of mice was fed green tea, another received white tea and a control group was given no treatment at all. Still others were given either green or white tea in combination with Sulindac. The mice that got nothing developed an average of about 30 tumors each. The mice that drank green tea had an average of 17 tumors each; those that drank white tea had an average of 13 tumors. The most dramatic results came from mice that were given both Sulindac *and* white tea: each averaged six tumors or only one-sixth of the number of cancers in untreated mice.

If the results of this study can be replicated in humans, it suggests that a combination of green or white tea with a NSAID, could dramatically reduce the risk for certain cancers of the colon.

Despite the dramatic results that regular and heavy aspirin use has shown in reducing the risk of advanced colon cancer, the side effects (including gastric bleeding and ulcers) can be serious and sometimes fatal. Another promising aspect of this study is that it suggests that smaller doses of aspirin or another drug could be equally effective in combination with tea. And those who cannot tolerate NSAIDs at all could receive the same protection the drugs afford without the dangerous side effects.

Optimal daily dose: 2,000 mg

Other nutrients useful for preventing colorectal cancer

Selenium

Selenium, another basic nutrient against cancer and specifically important against colorectal cancer, is a trace metal well known as a cancer fighter. Men and women who had taken selenium supplements (200 micrograms) for 10 years had significantly lower risks for several other cancers, including colorectal cancer, than those taking a placebo.

Another study pooled results from three clinical studies, comprising 1,700 patients who had had surgery on cancerous polyps in the colon, confirmed that selenium is effective at combating colorectal cancer. The researchers checked the selenium blood levels of all the patients and found that those with the highest levels had a significantly reduced risk of colon cancer recurrence than those with the lowest levels.

Probiotics

Numerous lab studies show that probiotics not only promote general gastrointestinal health but also can protect against colorectal cancer.

Adding beneficial bacteria to your intestinal tract through probiotics enhances immune function, helps make nutrients from food and supplements available to your body and helps flush toxins from your gastrointestinal (GI) tract.

Since nearly 70 percent of immune function in the human body takes place in the colon, the immune boosting influence of multi-strain probiotics (including *lactobacillus acidophilus* and *bifidobacterium* strain) slows or stops the growth of tumors in the GI tract.

Use a high-quality multi-strain probiotic product. The best require refrigeration to ensure the "good" bacteria you are re-introducing to your digestive tract are alive and potent.

While organic yogurt might be helpful as a food, its probiotic levels are generally too low to be effective in cancer prevention.

Dosage: Take according to manufacturer's instruction. Keep refrigerated.

In Summary

- Early detection is the key to defeating colorectal cancer. Have a screening every 10 years starting at age 50, earlier and more often if you have a family history of colorectal cancer.

- Maintain a healthy weight and exercise daily.

- The more vegetables and fruits in your diet, the less the likelihood you have of developing colorectal cancer. Adding certain supplements will help protect against the disease.

CHAPTER 20

Hormonally Related Cancers: Breast and Prostate

When I speak of hormonally-related cancers, I'm primarily talking about breast and prostate cancer, although several other types of cancer fall into this category, including ovarian, uterine, cervical, testicular, thyroid and osteosarcoma (a type of hormonally-related cancer that originates in the bones).

Breast and prostate cancers are the most common types of cancer in the U.S., after skin cancer.

We'll go into breast and prostate cancers separately, but there is a very important commonality among all types of hormonally-related cancer: many, if not most, are preventable.

Hormonally-related cancers are caused by:

1. Environmental toxins

2. Lifelong estrogen exposure

3. Genetics

4. Poor diet

5. Obesity

6. Sedentary lifestyle

7. Smoking

You've read the earlier chapters on cancer, so it's probably no surprise to you than these hormonally-related cancers are closely linked to diet, obesity and sedentary lifestyle with an important additional twist: they are also linked to the air we breathe, the water we drink, the clothing we wear and even the shampoos, soaps, makeup and cleaning products we use.

What are hormones?

Hormones are the chemical messengers of the body that transport signals from one cell to another. Hormones manufactured by the ovaries, testes, thyroid, pituitary glands, adrenal glands, pancreas and many other organs travel through the bloodstream to give instructions to the cells how to do their work. For example, insulin is a hormone produced by the pancreas that tells the cells how to use glucose for energy. Hormones are essential for growth and development, reproduction, digestion, energy levels and many other functions.

Estrogen, which is essential to our discussion in this chapter, is produced by the ovaries, adrenal glands and to a small degree, even male testes. These are the primary sex hormones in women that govern the onset of puberty, menstruation, sexual function, pregnancy, perimenopause and menopause. In men, the small amounts of estrogen naturally produced play a role in balancing hormones in general.

All hormones work on a "key and lock" system, meaning the hormone must fit itself into a receptor site on the cells for which they are meant in order for its function to occur within the cell. This is important when we look at hormonally–related cancers because excess amounts of hormones that cannot find receptors (there are no locks for the keys to fit into) circulate throughout the body, causing a variety of serious problems, including cancer.

Hormones are extremely powerful substances, so even a miniscule excess amount of a hormone can result in profound effects on the body, as we are about to learn.

Excess estrogen is the enemy in all hormonally-related cancers. I'll go into the details later, but it's important for you to know now that estrogens in the environment—which includes in your food, medicines, personal care and household cleaning products, even your furniture and car—all contribute to excess "unopposed" estrogen in your body. These false estrogen molecules can act just like estrogen, and sometimes can unlock cells, mimicking estrogen and all or some of its functions, usually not to your benefit. Some environmental estrogens cannot find cells to unlock, so they float around in the bloodstream, creating their own unique forms of havoc, including cancer. Those free estrogens also hide in fat cells, increasing the problem if you are overweight.

Breast cancer

About one in eight American women will develop invasive breast cancer in her lifetime. An estimated 232,000 new cases of invasive breast cancer will be diagnosed in 2013, according to the American Cancer Society's projections and nearly 40,000 American women will die of breast cancer.

Ductal carcinoma in situ (DCIS), a very early form of breast cancer that some experts now argue may not even be a true cancer, will be diagnosed in somewhat more than 64,000 women.

Men can get also get breast cancer, although it is 100 times less common than in women, with about 2,240 new cases expected in 2013.

In recent years, the cancer rates among women under 40 have increased, in my estimation because of exposure to environmental estrogens (I'll talk more about that soon). Younger women with breast cancer are more likely to die because many physicians dismiss their fears when they find breast lumps.

A woman with invasive breast cancer today has an 83.5 percent chance of surviving for five years. Forty years ago, she had a 75 percent chance of living five more years. In the 1970s, more than

60 percent of women diagnosed with breast cancer died within ten years, while the ten-year survival rate is now 77 percent. While these odds seem pretty good, the bigger concern is the increasing number of women diagnosed with breast cancer. The medical industry says it is because of increased awareness, earlier detection through mammograms and effective treatment. The wisdom of mammograms and radiation and chemotherapy are highly questionable in my mind, since they actually injure the body and deliberately expose it to cancer-causing radiation.

A thermal imaging method called a thermogram is an excellent non-invasive alternative to a mammogram that uses no radiation. Thermograms essentially measure heat in the human body and delineate "hot spots" where there is any kind of abnormal growth. They can show the earliest beginnings of tumors and abnormal growth of blood vessels, giving patients the opportunity to makes lifestyle corrections that can change the abnormality as long as ten years before it becomes cancerous. Thermograms are rarely covered by medical insurance, but the cost is not onerous, usually in the neighborhood of $100.

Thermograms are prediagnostic, even for women with dense breasts.

Ultrasounds can also be considered, especially for women with dense breasts and MRIs can also be effective, but they are expensive and unlikely to be covered by insurance unless you already have a diagnosis of breast cancer.

It's interesting to note that the breast cancer rate began dropping in 2000 and dropped a substantial seven percent from 2002 to 2003. It is not coincidental that this was the exact time frame when many women stopped taking Premarin and other synthetic hormone replacement (HRT) therapies after the Women's Health Initiative proved that these drugs greatly increase the risk of breast cancer. Since 2003, the breast cancer rates have remained stable.

Lifetime estrogen exposure is an important element in the hormonally-related cancer puzzle. Voluminous research shows that a woman's breast cancer risk increases the more estrogen a woman experiences in her lifetime (whether from the estrogen produced by her own body or in other ways, including HRT, birth control pills, pregnancies or xenoestrogens—those estrogen-like compounds found in food and many substances with which we all come into contact on a daily basis. I'll go into xenoestrogens in great depth later in this chapter.).

Genetics

Somewhere between 5 and 10 percent of breast cancers are the result of inherited genetic tendencies from genetic mutations known as BRCA-1 and BRCA-2 that also increase the risk of uterine, ovarian, cervical, pancreatic and colon cancers. Some women who have several close relatives with breast cancer have opted for gene testing to determine if they have the gene mutations that increase their lifetime risk of breast cancer alone by nearly eight-fold.

For men who get breast cancer, it is not clear if or how genetic mutations are a factor.

Although you might possess a gene that predisposes you to breast cancer, it is not inevitable that you will develop the disease. The new science of epigenetics shows us that changes in lifestyle, most notably in diet, can actually neutralize genetic tendencies for a variety of diseases, including preventing an estimated 50 percent of all breast cancers.

Prostate cancer

One in six American men will be diagnosed with prostate cancer sometime in his life. It is the most common cancer among American men and, happily, one of the most treatable.

An estimated 238,000 new cases of prostate cancer are expected in the U.S. in 2013, similar to the number of cases of invasive breast cancer. About 30,000 men die of prostate cancer a year.

African American men are almost twice as likely to die of prostate cancer as Caucasian men, although the long-term survival rates are good in almost all cases. The five-year survival rate for men with prostate cancer today is nearly 100 percent, compared to only 69 percent 40 years ago. Nearly 93 percent will survive for 15 years as opposed to only 69 percent 40 years ago.

Prostate cancer is commonly diagnosed by a blood test called the PSA (prostate specific antigen) or through a digital rectal exam that indicates enlargement of the prostate. There are usually no symptoms in the early stages and, even in more advanced stages, the most common symptom is a slowed or weakened urinary stream and the need to urinate more often, especially at night. However, these symptoms are more often caused by a mild condition called benign prostatic hyperplasia (BPH) or simply enlarged prostate.

Conventional medicine links excess testosterone to prostate cancer, but that really doesn't make much sense, especially in view of the fact that prostate cancer risk *increases* as a man ages, when we also know that a man's testosterone levels decline at the same time. Instead, experts in hormones and aging like the late John R. Lee, M.D., author of numerous books, including *Hormone Balance for Men,* theorizes that men's levels of progesterone decline with age, allowing estriol, one of the three main types of estrogen, to become dominant in their bodies and promoting malignant cell growth.

I think the early detection of prostate cancer through almost universal annual blood screening is probably the reason why prostate cancer now has such a high survival rate.

Genetics

While there is no specific gene yet identified linked with prostate cancer, about 20 percent of men with prostate cancer have family members who have had the disease, so it's a fair guess that there is a genetic component.

Environmental toxins

Our modern world is riddled with environmental toxins that are strong elements of today's hormonally-related cancers.

Probably the most important of these are substances known as endocrine disruptors. Endocrine disruptors damage hormone production and usage, negatively effecting reproductive, growth and developmental, metabolic, neurological and immunological health in humans and wildlife.

Endocrine disruptors are everywhere. They are in our water, our food, the containers in which our foods are packaged, prescription drugs, personal care products, household cleaning products, cars, garden and lawn care products and even in the diapers our babies wear and the shirts we put on our backs.

Among the most harmful hormone disruptors are:

- Dioxins and PCBs—highly toxic chemicals that are largely the result many manufacturing processes, including industrial waste incineration, bleaching of pulp and paper, chemical manufacturing, industrial runoff, residential oil furnaces, smoking and even backyard garden waste burning; all dioxins cause cancer in humans

- DDT—pesticide, which was fortunately banned in 1972, but is still present in many human tissues

- Pesticides and herbicides of many types

- Phenols like bisphenol-A, found in lightweight hard plastics

- Phthlates—found in hardened plastic

- POPs (persistent organic pollutants) often used as pesticides that accumulate in fatty tissues and are working their way up the food chain

- Heavy metals like arsenic, lead, cadmium and mercury found increasingly in our food supply

Xenoestrogens

These specific hormone disruptors act like estrogen in the body, which makes them even more dangerous as cancer-causing substances. They originate outside the human body (from the Greek root word "xeno") in everything from environmental toxins to plant foods.

Remember the key and lock analogy I made earlier in this chapter? When there is excess estrogen in the human body (male or female, young or not), this "unopposed estrogen" causes trouble by circulating around the body, keys without the locks to open and then unlocking the wrong things, including signaling mechanisms that tell cells to live a normal cellular life and die when their time comes. Cancer—wild, uncontrolled cell growth —is at least partly the result of damaged or aging cells that don't die when their normal life cycle comes to an end.

This excess estrogen has been scientifically validated as a cause of hormonally-related cancers, perhaps even the major cause of these deadly diseases.

Hormone-laden meats, eggs and dairy products are among the xenoestrogens to which almost all of us are exposed on a daily basis. Estrogen is fed to conventionally-raised cattle and chickens to increase meat, milk and egg production. Of course, you are what you eat, so those hormones are passed along to all of us.

The prevalence of hormones in our meat-and milk-streams certainly contribute to or directly cause "precocious puberty," a newly-minted medical term that describes breast growth in little girls as young as one-year old, early puberty, the growing incidences of infertility and erectile dysfunction, the epidemic of "man boobs", the widespread nature of prostate cancer and the rising incidence of breast cancer among younger women. All of these are related to a lifetime of excess estrogen that becomes toxic to our bodies.

Action list

Food

It is impossible to avoid endocrine disruptors and xenoestrogens. They are in the very air we breathe and the water we drink. However, there is a great deal we can to do protect ourselves and our families.

Here a big one you can do right now:

Add cruciferous vegetables to your diet every single, day without fail. Broccoli, cauliflower, Brussels sprouts, cabbage and all of the other cruciferous vegetables have been shown to help neutralize that excess estrogen.

Diet is crucial, not only foods that help neutralize xenoestrogens, but eating clean food to begin with. The message is the same for hormonally-related cancers, other cancers and overall excellent health:

- Eat clean meat (hormone and antibiotic-free organic meats)

- Eat clean fish (wild caught only)

- Eat clean dairy (organic and from antibiotic-free and hormone-free cows and goats)

- Eat lots of low glycemic index vegetables, particularly cruciferous vegetables that have been shown to have hormonally-related cancer preventive properties.

- Maintain an appropriate body weight to help keep hormonal levels steady and prevent the accumulation of excess estrogen in fat tissue. Congratulate yourself if you shed excess pounds, but realize that the estrogens that accumulated in those fat tissues are now circulating throughout your body, so those cruciferous vegetables become even more important.

Clean your house

Common household items are teeming with hormone disruptors. These poisons are in your soap, shampoo, makeup,

IS YOUR HOUSE "CLEAN"?

Here are a few some of my favorite ways to "clean house" and minimize your exposure to hormone disruptors and xeno-estrogens:

- Choose chlorine-free products and unbleached paper products including diapers, tampons, menstrual pads, toilet paper, paper towels, and coffee filters.

- Avoid all synthetic pesticides, herbicides, and fungicides.

- Use filtered water for drinking and bathing to avoid chlorine.

- Do not leave plastic containers, especially drinking water, in the sun or inside your car to prevent the off-gassing of the BPA into the water. Better yet, don't buy water in plastic bottles. Use stainless steel or glass containers with home-filtered water.

- Do not microwave food in plastic containers. Better yet, don't microwave food at all since it destroys nutrients.

- Avoid the use of plastic wrap to cover food for storing or microwaving. Use glass or ceramics whenever possible to store food.

- Use chemical free, biodegradable laundry and household cleaning products whenever possible.

- Use chemical-free soaps, shampoo, conditioner, moisturizers, toothpastes and other personal care products.

- Avoid cosmetics and creams that have toxic chemicals and estrogenic ingredients such as parabens, sodium laurate and stearal konium chloride (Beware: these can hide under a variety of names.).

- Minimize your exposure to nail polish and nail polish removers.

- Use naturally-based fragrances. Essential oils are a good alternative.

- Read the labels on condoms and diaphragm gels. Many contain carcinogens.

- Minimize X-rays whenever possible.

- Find a highly qualified environmental dentist to remove mercury-based fillings.

- Be aware of noxious gases from cleaning products (especially bleach and ammonia), carpets, particle board furniture, paint, copiers and printers and at the gas pump.

- Finally and most important: become a detective. Read labels diligently. Know what you are putting in and on your body. Deeply research what you use in your home and garden. It's a challenge, but you can clean up your life and your diet and minimize your risk of hormonally-related cancers.

deodorant, toilet paper, cookware, baby toys, carpets, furniture, cotton clothing, plastic wrap, car interiors, microwave ovens and practically everything you use to clean your house and yard and more.

Do you have any plastic in your home or yard? Who doesn't? It's nearly impossible to avoid. Virtually all soft or hard plastic is carcinogenic. When I think of our children and grandchildren chewing on soft plastic toys, I cringe.

An interesting side story here: a friend of mine decided she would not acquire any new plastic in her home for one year. She gave it up for impossible after just two months: her organic meat came wrapped in plastic; the organic pest control products she bought for her garden came only in plastic containers, shipped plastic-wrapped in boxes padded with bubble wrap; wine bottles had plastic corks; organic shampoos and even top quality supplements came in plastic bottles. She threw up her hands in frustration. It simply is not possible to banish plastic from our lives, but there is a great deal we can do to regain control and live cleaner, healthier lives.

Supplements

Here is a short list of supplements to add to the supplements mentioned at the beginning of this section that have specific properties to protect you against hormonally-related cancers.

Natural progesterone

Excess estrogen can be balanced by creams made from natural progesterone often obtained in very exact dosages from a compounding pharmacy, formulated specifically for an individual's needs. Again, always check with your doctor before using these.

Be very careful when you get you progesterone cream that it is *natural,* not synthetic. Natural progesterone cream is made from plant steroids found in wild yams. It is identical to the progesterone produced by women's ovaries.

Synthetic progesterones like Provera or medroxyprogesterone, have been scientifically proven to increase the risk of hormonally-related cancers, heart disease, stroke and Alzheimer's disease as well as depression, abnormal menstrual flow, fluid retention and nausea.

The only side effect associated with natural progesterone is the possibility of an altered menstrual cycle for women who are perimenopausal.

Dosage: According to your doctor's recommendation.

DIM (diindolylmethane)

This is the powerful substance found in cruciferous vegetables that has been shown over and over again to protect against hormonally-related cancers. (And no, taking DIM doesn't mean you don't have to eat your broccoli!) DIM + I3C (Indole-3-Carbinol) change the ratio of 2-hydroxy estrone to 16-hydroxy estrone. The more 2 and the less 16, the better. A simple blood test can check for this.

DIM helps balance estrogen as well as increasing production of healthy estrogens and lowering the levels of harmful free estrogens. For people who have been diagnosed with breast cancer, DIM has been shown to slow breast cancer cell growth and it works well with the oft-prescribed cancer companion drug tamoxifen as well as slowing or stopping the growth of blood supply that feeds cancerous tumors.

Optimal daily dose: DIM—200 mg; I3C—4,000 mg

Soy isoflavones

These plant steroids contain a natural plant estrogen that is 500 times weaker than human estrogen. Isoflavones, the active ingredients in soy products, actually compete with harmful free estrogens and bind to those receptor sites (the locks), effectively blocking strong xenoestrogens from attaching themselves to the cells.

By blocking the ability of harmful estrogens to communicate with the cells, soy phytoestrogens help reduce the estrogen load of the body.

Research shows soy isoflavones reduce the risk of several types of cancer including hormonally-related cancers and help relieve menopausal symptoms such as hot flashes.

Soy isoflavones also contain a substance called genistein, an antioxidant that controls the formation of new blood vessels to feed existing tumors.

If you are using soy as a food, use only *fermented* soy products like miso, tempeh, natto and traditionally-prepared soy sauce. These healthy fermented products are more biologically available to the human body. Unfermented products like tofu and soy milk contain a variety of harmful "anti-nutrients" that can actually increase estrogen levels in the human body and contribute to the risk of hormonally-related cancers.

In addition, unless you have a certified organic soy product, you can be assured it comes from a genetically modified seed, since 90 percent of all soy grown worldwide is now genetically modified and carries with it unknown health risks.

It's best to get your soy isoflavones as a supplement from a certified organic source. Use only fermented soy.

Optimal daily dose: 400 mg

Calcium D-Glucarate

A potent detoxification aid studied at the University of Texas M.D. Anderson Cancer Center, AMC Cancer Center, Ohio State University, and Memorial Sloan-Kettering Cancer Center of New York, calcium d-glucarate promotes cell health of the liver, prostate, lung, breast and colon. Derived from fruits and vegetables, calcium d-glucarate moderates beta-glucuronidase, which supports the elimination of toxins, endogenous compounds and environmental substances responsible for abnormal cell growth.

Actually, one dose of calcium d-glucarate is equivalent to 82 pounds of fresh fruits and vegetables. Because of its powerful action on the body, calcium d-glucarate may prove helpful against the development of certain tumors. Estrogen dominance, which interferes with normal hormone balance, is associated with fibroids, endometriosis, and premenstrual syndrome.

By inhibiting estrogen receptor sites, calcium d-glucarate prevents the recirculating of toxins and free estrogen. When this happens, estrogen stays bound to its water-soluble bond, and the total toxic load on the body is drastically reduced.

Optimal daily dose: 400 mg

DHEA (*dehydroepiandrosterone*)

This master hormone, produced by the adrenal glands, instructs the body to produce more (or less) estrogen and testosterone. Sometimes called the "fountain of youth" nutrient, animal studies showed individuals with less gray hair, shinier coats, and most important, lower risk of hormonally-related cancers and stronger immune systems than animals that did not receive DHEA.

Research on DHEA is mixed, with some studies showing DHEA protects against breast cancer cell growth and blocking the estrogen receptors (locks) on cells while others contradict that finding.

If you're considering taking DHEA or any other supplements, be sure to consult your health care provider.

Optimal daily dose: 10 mg

Melatonin

This hormone produced by the pineal gland, is best known for regulating our sleep/wake cycles. It is produced in complete darkness, a good reason to keep your bedroom as dark as possible.

Melatonin also awakens a gene called P53, the gene that tells cells when they are too old or too damaged and instructs them to die. When P53 goes to sleep, old and damaged cells can grow out of control and become malignant.

Melatonin also blocks those estrogen "locks" on cells, keeping dangerous estrogens from delivering their deadly message as well as protecting against cortisol (stress) induced cellular damage and non-estrogen related cellular changes that lead to breast cancer.

Melatonin is so powerful it is often used in addition to chemotherapy for those who choose conventional approaches to cancer.

Optimal daily dose: 3 mg taken at bedtime

Alzheimer's, Dementia and Age-Related Cognitive Decline

CHAPTER 21

What Are Mental Decline, Dementia and Alzheimer's Disease?

Our American culture preprograms people to believe that cognitive function declines as we age. There are countless jokes, even television sitcoms that exploit Grandma leaving the car keys in the freezer or Grandpa getting lost on the way home from the grocery or groping for a word or name.

While we may chuckle at the foibles of the elderly, it's not funny when it happens to us or those we love.

Perhaps we laugh because we are uncomfortably aware that we may share this fate in a few years or a few decades.

Perhaps it also because our culture tends to dismiss the wisdom of our elders, unlike Native American societies or indigenous cultures who live close to the Earth.

Perhaps it is also a self-fulfilling prophecy that the elderly start to become forgetful—or worse—and since we believe this will happen, it does.

There are approximately 45 million Americans who are age 65 or older. That number is expected to nearly double by 2050.

One in eight older Americans has Alzheimer's and that number increases to half of all of those over the age of 85. Alzheimer's is the sixth leading cause of death in the U.S. and more than 5.2 million people today are living with the disease.

One in three seniors dies from Alzheimer's or dementia, so you can see it is a serious national, personal and family problem.

Death from Alzheimer's increased 68 percent between 2000 and 2010, while death rates dropped from all other dread diseases, primarily heart disease and cancer. Fifteen million Americans provide care for someone with Alzheimer's or other dementia and we spend another $200 billion for paid caregivers. That cost is expected to rise to $1.2 trillion by 2050 when the prevalence of the disease will have increased by 40 percent.

Sadly, conventional medicine has no treatment for Alzheimer's and dementia, except the relatively rare reversible forms of dementia I mention later in this chapter. The U.S. Food and Drug Administration (FDA) has approved five drugs for Alzheimer's that *may* temporarily slow the progression of the disease in some people. Some doctors will recommend brain scans to identify the amount of a beta amyloid, a protein related to Alzheimer's, to confirm diagnosis, but a diagnosis is pretty much pointless since there is no real treatment. In other words, conventional medicine puts little credence in the concept of preventing Alzheimer's and even less in the chance of slowing or even reversing it.

Mild cognitive impairment (MCI)

As I've mentioned in previous chapters, we know that cells deteriorate with age. Over time, the body's ability to reproduce and create new cells that are exact copies of the previous ones begins to decline. If new cells are not precisely the same as their parent cells, cells don't function as well as cells did in earlier generations.

In simple terms, many bodily functions do decline with age, and brain function is among them. Older people may be forgetful, lose their ability to maintain focus and have diminished ability to solve problems and multitask, something that is frequently called executive function today. Studies suggest 10 to 20 percent of the population over the age of 65 has some level of mild cognitive impairment (MCI).

Factors in MCI, also known as age-related cognitive decline:

- oxidative stress and free radical damage
- chronic low-level inflammation
- declining hormone levels
- excess body weight
- poor diet
- lifestyle
- social network
- genetics
- dysfunction of the lining of the blood vessels

What's normal, what's not

Probably many of my readers are wondering, "Do I have cognitive impairment?"

If you're reading this book, my answer would be, "Probably not."

MCI is not the same as dementia and does not mean that cognitive impairment will lead to dementia or Alzheimer's. In fact, only 10 to 15 percent of cases of MCI develop into some form of dementia. The key is that MCI does not cause any alteration to a person's daily activities.

As we age, there are detectable changes in the brain: its weight drops by about 10 percent at age 80; blood flow diminishes; neurons and dendritic connections die or become impaired and nerve functions slow.

However, the human brain has great reserve capacity and brain cells can not only regenerate, they can grow new cells and new dendrites, those finger-like connections to other cells, literally forming alternate "electrical" pathways for thoughts

COGNITIVE IMPAIRMENT SELF-TEST

Here are a few questions to ask yourself and those closest to you, who may be able to give you a more objective assessment. Do you:

- Forget things more often over the past year or two?

- Forget appointments, social engagements or birthdays?

- Lose your train of thought or concentration during conversations or while reading a book or watching a movie?

- Feel increasingly overwhelmed by the need to make decisions, plan steps to complete a task or interpret instructions?

- Have some trouble finding your way around familiar places?

- Become more impulsive or show poor judgment beyond your normal patterns?

If you answered "yes" to any of these questions, ask your family and friends if they have noticed changes. Be open to their answers.

and other brain functions. Think of an electrical system. If the system has multiple circuits and one or two circuits go bad, the electricity can reroute itself around the damaged circuits and still continue to function. The human brain works much the same way.

Dementia

Dementia is an umbrella term for memory loss that includes Alzheimer's, but also includes a variety of other types of mental decline, some of which are reversible.

It's also an umbrella term for a bundle of symptoms including

COMMON SIGNS AND SYMPTOMS OF DEMENTIA

- Memory loss
- Impaired judgment
- Difficulties with abstract thinking
- Faulty reasoning
- Inappropriate behavior
- Loss of communication skills
- Disorientation to time and place
- Gait, motor and balance problems
- Neglect of personal care and safety
- Hallucinations, paranoia, agitation

Source: Helpguide.org

memory loss, personality change and impaired mental function that result either from a disease or injury (brain trauma).

If you've noticed a decline in communication, learning ability, short-term memory and problem solving (quickly or over a year or two), those are strong signs of dementia or Alzheimer's.

Shrinkage of brain mass and damage to the nerve cells of the brain are the simple symptoms of dementia, but those are symptoms, not causes, as we'll see in the coming pages.

Alzheimer's disease

Alzheimer's is the most common form of dementia, accounting for 60 to 80 percent of all cases. It is called "progressive" because it worsens over time. It is most commonly found in people over the age of 60, but there has been a recent surge in the number of people with early-onset forms of Alzheimer's, most likely because of damaged genes, frequently the result of environmental factors.

Diagnosis is an imprecise science, but it usually involves a basic neurological exam, testing coordination and balance, lab tests that will show if dementia is due to vitamin deficiencies and a mental function test. In recent years, CT and PET scans and MRIs have increasingly been used to identify unique Alzheimer's-related changes in the brain.

People with Alzheimer's usually decline over a period of years, most commonly seven to 10 years. Many doctors will assume a diagnosis of Alzheimer's, although there are reversible forms of dementia due to nutritional deficiencies and injuries, so family members would do well to insist on detailed testing to determine the type of dementia that is present.

There a number of causes of Alzheimer's, some of them quite surprising.

Genetics

Three forms of a gene called APOE have been associated with increased risk of Alzheimer's as have others known as SORL1, CLU, CR1, PICALM and TREM2. These genes only represent risk factors for Alzheimer's, not a certainty that a person will develop the disease, even if the genes have been inherited from both parents. Only about 5 percent of Alzheimer's cases are believed to be genetic.

In any case, since scientists now almost universally agree that lifestyle and environment can reduce or even reverse these genetic risks, the new science of epigenetics once again comes into play.

Heart disease and stroke

Heart disease, stroke and chronic high blood pressure are linked to Alzheimer's though a condition called chronic brain hypoperfusion (CBH), more simply, decreased blood flow to the brain. Decreased blood flow to the brain has also been linked to the formation of the characteristic plaques and tangles in brain tissues that disrupt brain activity and define Alzheimer's.

Type 2 diabetes

Alzheimer's has been called "diabetes of the brain" in the sense that brain cells depend on glucose for their function, so the impaired glucose function of Type 2 diabetes causes damage to brain cells. Healthy brain function is also the result of a delicate dance of multiple brain chemicals. High blood sugar also causes inflammation that may damage brain cells. Insulin imbalances can harm these chemical reactions needed for correct mental function.

Chlamydia

This type of common pneumonia bacteria (*Chlamydia pneumonaie*), not to be confused with the sexually transmitted disease, has been closely linked to Alzheimer's. This insidious bacteria has also been linked to heart disease and atherosclerosis. Researchers have found the *Chlamydia* bacteria in the brains of people who died of late-onset Alzheimer's and not in the ones who did not suffer from the disease, indicating the bacteria has a role in Alzheimer's.

Helicobacter pylori bacteria

This bacteria has been found as a cause of nearly all stomach ulcers and it has a link to Alzheimer's as well. There is some speculation that infection with *H. pylori* stomach ulcers might block the absorption of vitamin B_{12}, bringing on a form of dementia connected to deficiency of that vital brain nutrient. *H. pylori* also has a link to Type 2 diabetes and atherosclerosis, both of which increase the risk of Alzheimer's.

Herpes virus

The herpes simplex virus Type 1 (HSV-1), which causes cold sores, is present in 90 percent of all adults. Research has recently shown that HSV-1 has been found in the "hallmark" beta amyloid protein that is diagnostic for Alzheimer's. They've also discovered the herpes virus had a hiding place where it can evade the immune system for decades: the neurons of the brain, where it incubates for years and causes persistent brain inflammation and occasional cold sore outbreaks. Canadian researchers have concluded that HSV-1 is a major cause of beta-amyloid plaques and they suggest that the discovery of a vaccine against HSV-1 could also be a major breakthrough in preventing Alzheimer's.

Nitrates in food and agriculture

Nitrates are among the toxic substances, present in our everyday life, that are hard to avoid. A Brown University researcher has termed us "the nitrosamine generation" because of the presence of nitrates in:

• Preserved foods: ham, bacon, lunch meats, hotdogs, sausages and more

• Other foods, including charbroiled meat, ground beef, salted, pickled canned and smoked fish, beer, aged cheeses, nonfat dried milk and foods fried at high temperatures

• Tobacco smoke

• Rubber products

• Pesticides

• Some cosmetics

• Water leeched from agricultural applications into food and drinking water

The connection between nitrosamines and cancer has been well established, but the connection with Alzheimer's is lesser known. The Brown researchers theorize that nitrates and nitrosamines damage DNA and destroy brain cells. Nitrates may also trigger the liver to produce toxins that destroy brain cells.

Aluminum

The link between Alzheimer's and aluminum, found in cookware, antacids, soda cans and antiperspirant deodorants, is controversial and spotty. For more than 30 years, scientists have known that aluminum has been found in the brains of people with Alzheimer's. Some studies show that people who use aluminum cookware and antiperspirants containing aluminum chlorhydrate have a higher risk for Alzheimer's, while other studies counter that theory.

I recommend avoiding products that contain aluminum for safety's sake. There are plenty of alternatives.

Aspartame

The link between Alzheimer's and aspartame is also controversial. Aspartame is found in the popular artificial sweeteners Equal and Sweet 'N Low and in a wide array of soft drinks and other artificially sweetened foods and beverages. Aspartame is made up of three chemicals: aspartic acid, phenylalanine, and methanol. Aspartic acid is one of many neurotransmitters (brain chemical) that feeds neurons and enhances brain health, until we get too much, when it kills neurons by allowing too much calcium into the cells. It has been linked to Alzheimer's as well as a variety of other neurological diseases.

Radiation exposure

Radiation kills cells and when it is used for therapeutic reasons, for example to treat malignant tumors, it also effects nearby cells. That's why it is so important to minimize your exposure to routine X-rays, mammograms and CT scans and to make a careful analysis before engaging in cancer-related radiation treatments, especially if they involve the brain, head or neck because Alzheimer's could be a side effect.

Other types of dementia

Aside from Alzheimer's, let's talk about other forms of dementia. Although there are some reversible forms of dementia, most types, like Alzheimer's, are irreversible and progressive, meaning the person with the disease will deteriorate over time. Modern medicine doesn't provide much in the way of pharmaceuticals to delay the progression of these diseases, television advertising to the contrary.

Genetics

There can be genetic components for all types of dementia, but scientists are increasingly recognizing epigenetic factors of environmental and lifestyle factors that are also important elements.

Lewy bodies

This type of dementia, making up 20 percent or more of cases, results from some distinctive clumps of protein found in the brains of people with the disease. Symptoms are similar to Alzheimer's and other types of dementia, with one unique element: people with this type of dementia tend to rapidly fluctuate between times of clear thinking and confusion. They are also prone to hallucinations, tremors and rigidity similar to Parkinson's disease.

Vascular dementia

This type of dementia is the result of brain damage because of impaired blood flow to the brain, often because of a heart attack or stroke or even high blood pressure. Vascular dementia usually starts suddenly.

Traumatic brain injury

Caused by a blow to the head and bleeding within the brain cavity, traumatic brain injuries can cause dementia as we've seen in recent years with the publicity attached to increasing rates of dementia among football players who experience repeated blows to the head as well as soldiers injured in combat.

Brain diseases

Parkinson's disease and Huntington's disease are known triggers for dementia and they usually begin around the ages of 30 and 40. Other diseases like Creutzfeld-Jakob (mad cow) and HIV can destroy brain cells and cause dementia, although they are not common. Sleep apnea, a distressingly common disease, which causes people to literally stop breathing several times a night, deprives the brain of oxygen and can also contribute to brain cell death and Alzheimer's.

Chemical exposures

Long-term association with various toxic chemicals can also cause dementia. Lead, pesticides, PCBs and particulate air pollution can permanently damage brain cells and cause dementia as can high levels of mercury in fish and mercury amalgam dental fillings.

Reversible forms of dementia

A number of conditions can cause dementia that can be reversed, including infections like meningitis, encephalitis, untreated syphilis and Lyme disease or immune disorders like leukemia as well as brain tumors.

Dementia can also be caused by nutritional deficiencies, including dehydration (simply not drinking enough water) and deficiencies of vitamins B_6 and B_{12} in the diet. Vitamin B_1 (thiamine) deficiency, common in alcoholics, is a cause of dementia as are abuse of alcohol and recreational drugs.

Reactions to medications or drug interactions have also been known to cause dementia as have poisoning from exposure to heavy metals, especially lead and pesticides, which, if exposure has not been long-term, may be reversible through the use of chelation therapy.

It can also be connected to a sudden decline in the flow of oxygen to the brain that can accompany a severe asthma attack, a heart attack or carbon monoxide poisoning.

If you or a loved one is experiencing symptoms of dementia, be sure your doctor considers the reversible causes of dementia.

Preventing Alzheimer's and other forms of dementia

Most of us have heard about the heart healthy effects of a Mediterranean diet rich in fruits, vegetables, olive oil and fish, and research also shows that it may lower the risk of cognitive decline by as much as 40 percent, according to Columbia University researchers.

Staying physically active *and* following a Mediterranean diet reduced the risk of Alzheimer's even more, said the same study, by 61 to 67 percent. The Fight Fat with Fat Diet, which is low in sugar and carbohydrates and high in natural and saturated fats, will have the same effects.

Research shows that this type of diet may:

- Slow cognitive decline in older adults

- Reduce the risk of mild cognitive impairment

- Reduce the risk of a heart attack progressing into Alzheimer's disease

Keys to preventing cognitive decline are:

Healthy diet. I've discussed this at length throughout this book and increasing evidence points to the preventive qualities of a healthy diet and proper weight in preventing virtually every disease mentioned in this book. This is also true for Alzheimer's and other forms of dementia. Plenty of omega-3 fatty acids, like those found in fatty fish like salmon and tuna, are also important for healthy brain cells. Green tea is also linked to brain health.

Regular exercise. The simple acts of movement and oxygenation of the blood help promote brain health by nourishing brain cells. Exercise also helps improve memory, reduce stress and improve mood. The Alzheimer's Research and Prevention Foundation says regular exercise reduces the risk of Alzheimer's by 50 percent. This means at least 30 minutes of aerobic exercise at least five times a week, two 15-minutes of strength training and some balance training.

Regular mental stimulation. The adage says, "Use it or lose it," and this seems to be particularly true for keeping memory intact. Do whatever challenges your brain: solve crossword puzzles or Sudoku, take a class at your community college, learn a new language, engage in enthusiastic discussion of ideas you find interesting, memorize a poem you love. The key here is to do something new and different to keep your brain sharp.

Quality sleep. Most of us need eight hours of sleep a night, but few of us get that much. Deep sleep and dreaming are important for keeping your productivity and creativity up to par. Keeping your body's natural rhythms intact and sleeping and waking at roughly the same time every day can go a long way toward supporting your brain and body functions. If your partner tells you that you snore, you should be checked for sleep apnea, which has been linked to Alzheimer's and may even be a sign of early-stage Alzheimer's.

Manage stress. We all have stress in our lives, but those toxic stress hormones have been shown to lead to shrinkage of the hippocampus, the memory center of the brain, slowing nerve growth and increasing the risk of Alzheimer's. Do yoga, listen to music, take time alone, meditate, attend spiritual services to help keep toxic stress at bay. There are many excellent stress management books available. Glean some helpful techniques and reclaim your health.

Have an active social life. Numerous studies show that people who are the most socially engaged and who create a wide network of friends and family have the lowest risk of cognitive decline. No friends and family? New to your area? Create some new networks. Join a class at the community college, go to church, volunteer at the local soup kitchen. Do whatever it takes to be engaged in your community and friends and family. You'll reap the benefits.

MY PRESCRIPTION FOR BRAIN HEALTH

Take a ballroom dancing class

You'll have to learn something new.

You'll get some excellent aerobic exercise.

You'll laugh and reduce stress.

You'll meet new people.

You'll sleep better.

Five of the six preventive strategies in one fun activity. Not bad!

CHAPTER 22

The Salerno Solution Brain Health Supplement Program

The following list of supplements has been clinically proven to be effective in the prevention and treatment of Alzheimer's disease and, in some cases, forms of dementia and other memory loss.

Curcumin

I've mentioned curcumin several times in this book, because it is such a powerful preventer and treatment for a variety of diseases, including Alzheimer's. New studies show very clearly that this potent antioxidant can lower toxic beta amyloid protein levels and preserve brain cells and actually can stimulate the formation of new brain cells, especially in the hippocampus, the brain's memory center.

Optimal daily dose: 1,000 mg

Fish oil

Another almost universally effective supplement that I have to mention again in terms of Alzheimer's and dementia, fish has always been called "brain food" for good reason. The omega-3 fatty acids in fatty fish like salmon and tuna are essential to learning and memory. The DHA (docosahexaenoic acid) helps strengthen the fatty membrane around nerve cells as well as acting as an anti-inflammatory. Research shows it is more effective preventing the disease rather than the ability to slow progression of Alzheimer's once it has begun. DHA has also been shown to increase levels of a vital protein that is found in reduced levels in Alzheimer's patients.

Optimal daily dose: 2,000 mg

Choline

This essential nutrient for brain development is used by the brain in the manufacture of acetylcholine, to form memory. People with Alzheimer's have lower acetylcholine levels than those who do not have the disease, suggesting supplementation with choline may help prevent dementia.

Optimal daily dose: L-glycerol phosphoryl choline: 500 mg

B vitamins

This complex of several vitamins has been clinically shown to reduce brain shrinkage and to regulate levels of homocysteine, an amino acid found in the blood that, among other things, contributes to brain shrinkage and dementia. Studies show that the more B vitamins in the blood, the less homocysteine, and they can reverse brain shrinkage in Alzheimer's patients by 30 percent or more. All the B complex vitamins are important and B_{12} may have some particular properties to prevent and even reverse dementia.

Optimal daily dose: 1 B Complex 500

Magnesium

In people with early- to midstage Alzheimer's, the ones with the lowest ionized magnesium (active magnesium) levels were the ones with the most impaired cognitive function, particularly in the hippocampus or memory center of the brain. It is estimated that about 80 percent of Americans are magnesium deficient, so supplementation could be a good measure for overall health and for staving off dementia.

Optimal daily dose: 400 mg

Acetyl l-carnitine

This amino acid has been shown to protect nerves from damage and to increase attention span by as much as 50 percent in people with Alzheimer's as well as to slow down the deterioration associated with all types of dementia.

Optimal daily dose: 2 grams

Phosphatidylserine (PS)

This component of membranes that enclose brain cells strengthens cells and prevents damage or further damage. The small number of studies on PS suggests it is best used as a preventive to keep memory sharp and even to help regain short-term memory. It can also be effective in the early stages of Alzheimer's.

Optimal daily dose: 100 mg and up to 300 mg if memory loss and dementia are already taking place.

Coconut oil

There is no research yet on the brain-nourishing effects of coconut oil, but information widely circulated on the Internet suggests that the unique fats in coconut oil are converted into ketones by the liver and those ketones can be used as an alternative fuel by brain cells impaired by Type 2 diabetes. While this is very shaky scientifically, coconut oil is a healthy fat and there is no harm in adding it to the diet of someone showing signs of dementia.

Optimal daily dose: 2 tablespoons (can be used in cooking)

Coenzyme Q-10

I've mentioned Co Q-10 numerous times in this book because it is vital to cell health and improves a variety of degenerative diseases, including Alzheimer's. Early studies show supplementation may help slow down the progression of the disease.
Optimal daily dose: 1 mg per pound of body weight, i.e. a 150-pound person needs 150 mg

Vitamin D

You've heard about this super vitamin several times in the book as well. That's because it is so vitally important to so many bodily systems. New research shows that vitamin D_3 can actually clear the brain of those memory-destroying beta amyloid plaques, especially when combined with omega-3 fatty acids found in fish oil. Other research suggests that low levels of vitamin D in the blood increase the risk of Alzheimer's.
Optimal daily dose: 2,000 IU. Up to 5,000 IU if you have memory loss, plus 20 minutes a day in the sun with as much skin exposed as possible.

There are a few other supplements to consider because they have been shown to have some positive effects against Alzheimer's and dementia. Discuss your supplement regimen with your health care practitioner and determine what is best for you to prevent and/or slow the progression of memory loss, dementia and Alzheimer's. All are shown with optimal daily doses.

- L-Huperzine A: 400 mcg
- DMAE: 100 mg
- Vinpocetine: 15 mg
- Blueberry Extract: 100 mg
- Ashwagandha: 100 mg
- Berberine: 500–1,000 mg
- L-glutamine: 1,000 mg

CHAPTER 23

Conclusion

I know I've packed a huge amount of information into this modest book. I wish I could make it an encyclopedia because there is so much to share with you. That will come in other books.

Take some time with this book. Read, reread and digest the sections that pertain the most to you. Most importantly, really read the first section. Section 1 has the keys to disease prevention through simple lifestyle changes that you can make that will reward you with profound long-term improvements to your health.

Take it all in small bites. Bit by bit, you'll notice changes in your energy level, the disappearance of aches and pain, small digestive upsets and even your waistline.

If you have any of the diseases I mention in this book—heart disease, diabetes, cancer or memory impairment—in a few weeks you may begin to notice changes. What you won't notice is the heart disease that never develops, the Type 2 diabetes that you banished or the cancer or dementia that you escaped by making healthy lifestyle choices.

I realize that my recommendations are somewhat outside of the mainstream. My two decades of watching patients follow the Atkins protocols and my Fight Fat with Fat Diet show me that this lifestyle plans works.

Welcome to the journey toward vibrant health and long life!

References

Section 2: Preventing Heart Disease, Stroke and Hypertension

Crowe FL, Key TJ, Appleby PN, et al. Dietary fibre intake and ischaemic heart disease mortality: the European Prospective Investigation into Cancer and Nutrition-Heart study. *European Journal of Clinical Nutrition.* 2012 Aug;66(8):950–6.

Minihane, MA, Fish oil omega-3 fatty acids and cardio-metabolic health, alone or with statins. *European Journal of Clinical Nutrition* advance online publication, 13 February 2013; (2013).

Haast RA, Gustafson DR, Kiliaan AJ. Sex differences in stroke. *Journal of Cerebral Blood Flow Metabolism.* 2012 Dec;32(12):2100–7.

Dauchet L, Amouyel P, Hercberg S, Dallongeville J. Fruit and vegetable consumption and risk of coronary heart disease: a meta-analysis of cohort studies. *Journal of Nutrition.* 2006 Oct;136(10):2588–93.

Marik PE, Varon J. Omega-3 dietary supplements and the risk of cardiovascular events: a systematic review. *Clinical Cardiology.* 2009 Jul;32(7): 365–72. doi: 10.1002/clc.20604.

Watts GF, Playford DA, et al. Coenzyme Q(10) improves endothelial dysfunction of the brachial artery in Type II diabetes mellitus. *Diabetologia.* 2002 Mar;45(3):420–6.

Section 3: Preventing and Treating Type 2 Diabetes

www.idf.org/diabetesatlas/5e/Update2012

Gulve EA. Exercise and glycemic control in diabetes: benefits, challenges, and adjustments to pharmacotherapy. *Phys Ther.* 2008 Nov;88(11):1297–321. doi: 10.2522/ptj.20080114. Epub 2008 Sep 18.

Duclos M, Virally ML, Dejager S. Exercise in the management of type 2 diabetes mellitus: what are the benefits and how does it work? *Phys Sportsmed.* 2011 May;39(2):98–106. doi: 10.3810/psm.2011.05.1899.

Porasuphatana S, Suddee S, Nartnampong A, Konsil J, Harnwong B, Santaweesuk A. Glycemic and oxidative status of patients with type 2 diabetes mellitus following oral administration of alpha-lipoic acid: a randomized double-blinded placebo-controlled study. *Asia Pacific Journal of Clinical Nutrition.* 2012;21(1):12–21.

Stohs SJ, Miller H, Kaats GR. A review of the efficacy and safety of banaba (Lagerstroemia speciosa L.) and corosolic acid. *Phytotherapeutic Research.* 2012 Mar;26(3):317–24. doi: 10.1002/ptr.3664. Epub 2011 Nov 17.

Lecube A, Baena-Fustegueras JA, Fort JM, Pelegrí D, Hernández C, Simó R. Diabetes is the main factor accounting for hypomagnesemia in obese subjects. *PLoS One.* 2012;7(1):e30599. doi: 10.1371/journal.pone.0030599. Epub 2012 Jan 24.

Section 4: Preventing Cancer

www.cancer.org/acs/groups/content/@epidemiologysurveilance/documents/document/acspc-036845.pdf

http://seer.cancer.gov/statfacts/html/lungb.html

Manson MM, Farmer PB, Gescher A, Steward WP. Innovative agents in cancer prevention. *Recent Results in Cancer Research.* 2005;166:257–75.

Zhong X, Zhang C. Soy food intake and breast cancer risk: a meta-analysis. *Wei Sheng Yan Jiu.* 2012 Jul;41(4):670–6. [article in Chinese]

Psaltopoulou T, Kosti RI, Haidopoulos D, Dimopoulos M, Panagiotakos DB. Olive oil intake is inversely related to cancer prevalence: a systematic review and a meta-analysis of 13,800 patients and 23,340 controls in 19 observational studies. *Lipids Health Disease.* 2011 Jul 30;10:127. doi: 10.1186/1476-511X-10-127.

Giovannucci E, Stampfer MJ, Colditz GA, Hunter DJ, Fuchs C, Rosner BA, Speizer FE, Willett WC. Multi-vitamin use, folate, and colon cancer in women in the Nurses' Health Study. *Annals of Internal Medicine.* 1998 Oct 1;129(7): 517–24.

Holick, C. et al. Dietary carotenoids, serum beta-carotene, and retinol and risk of lung cancer in the alpha-tocopherol, beta-carotene cohort study. *American Journal of Epidemiology.* 2002. 156(6):536–47.

Hoffmann D, Hoffmann I, El-Bayoumy K. The less harmful cigarette: a controversial issue. a tribute to Ernst L. Wynder. *Chemical Res Toxicology.* 2001 Jul;14(7):767–90.

Peto R, Darby S, Deo H, Silcocks P, Whitley E, Doll R. Smoking, smoking cessation, and lung cancer in the UK since 1950: combination of national statistics with two case-control studies. *British Medical Journal.* 2000 Aug 5;321(7257):323–9.

Hashibe M, Morgenstern H, Cui Y, et al. Marijuana use and the risk of lung and upper aerodigestive tract cancers: results of a population-based case-control study. *Cancer Epidemiology, Biomarkers and Prevention.* 2006;15(10):1829–34.

Office on Smoking and Health (US), editors. The Health Consequences of Involuntary Exposure to Tobacco Smoke: A Report of the Surgeon General. Atlanta (GA): Centers for Disease Control and Prevention (US); 2006.

Oberg M, Jaakkola MS, Woodward A, Peruga A, Prüss-Ustün A. Worldwide burden of disease from exposure to second-hand smoke: a retrospective analysis of data from 192 countries. *Lancet.* 2011 Jan 8;377(9760):139–46.

Olivo-Marston SE, Yang P, Mechanic LE, et al. Childhood exposure to secondhand smoke and functional mannose binding lectin polymorphisms are associated with increased lung cancer risk. *Cancer Epidemiology Biomarkers & Prevention.* 2009 Dec;18(12):3375–83.

Jiang Q, Wong J, Fyrst H, Saba JD, Ames BN. gamma-Tocopherol or combinations of vitamin E forms induce cell death in human prostate cancer cells by interrupting sphingolipid synthesis. *Proceedings of the National Academy of Science USA.* 2004 Dec 21;101(51):17825–30. Epub 2004 Dec 13.

Rose DP, Connolley JM. Omega-3 fatty acids as cancer chemopreventive agents. *Pharmacology Therapies* 1999;83:217–44.

www.cancer.org/acs/groups/content/@epidemiologysurveilance/documents/document/acspc-036845.pdf

Yu MC, Yuan JM. Environmental factors and risk for hepatocellular carcinoma. *Gastroenterology.* 2004 Nov;127(5 Suppl 1):S72–8.

Egner PA, Wang JB, Zhu YR, et al. Chlorophyllin intervention reduces aflatoxin-DNA adducts in individuals at high risk for liver cancer. *Proceedings of the National Academy of Science USA.* 2001 Dec 4;98(25):14601–6.

Ron E. Cancer risks from medical radiation. *Health Physician.* 2003 Jul;85(1):47–59.

Chow WH, McLaughlin JK, Zheng W, Blot WJ, Gao YT. Occupational risks for primary liver cancer in Shanghai, China. *American Journal of Ind Medicine.* 1993 Jul;24(1):93–100.

Morales KH, Ryan L, Kuo TL, Wu MM, Chen CJ. Risk of internal cancers from arsenic in drinking water. *Environmental Health Perspectives.* 2000 Jul;108(7):655–61.

Oommen S, Anto RJ, Srinivas G, Karunagaran D. Allicin (from garlic) induces caspase-mediated apoptosis in cancer cells. *European Journal of Pharmacology.* 2004 Feb 6;485(1–3):97–103

Bustamante J, Lodge JK, et al. Alpha-lipoic acid in liver metabolism and disease. *Free Radical Biological Medicine.* 1998 Apr;24(6):1023–39

Miura D, Miura Y, Yagasaki K. Resveratrol inhibits hepatoma cell invasion by suppressing gene expression of hepatocyte growth factor via its reactive oxygen species-scavenging property. *Clinical Exp Metastasis.* 2004;21(5):445–51.

Imai K, Nakachi K. Cross sectional study of effects of drinking green tea on cardiovascular and liver diseases. *British Medical Journal.* 1995;310:693–696.

Hansen RD, Albieri V, Tjønneland A, et al. Effects of smoking and antioxidant micronutrients on risk of colorectal cancer. *Clinical Gastroenterology & Hepatology.* 2013 Apr;11(4):406–415.e3. Epub 2012 Nov 6.

Chao A, Thun MJ, Jacobs EJ, et al. Cigarette smoking and colorectal cancer mortality in the cancer prevention study II. *Journal of the National Cancer Institute.* 2000 Dec 6;92(23):1888–96.

Park Y, Hunter DJ, Spiegelman D, et al. Dietary fiber intake and risk of colorectal cancer: a pooled analysis of prospective cohort studies. *Journal of the American Medical Assn.* 2005 Dec 14;294(22):2849–57.

Park Y, Spiegelman D, Hunter DJ, et al. Intakes of vitamins A, C, and E and use of multiple vitamin supplements and risk of colon cancer: a pooled analysis of prospective cohort studies. *Cancer Causes Control.* 2010 Nov;21(11): 1745–57.

Gandini S, Boniol M, Haukka J, et al. Meta-analysis of observational studies of serum 25-hydroxyvitamin D levels and colorectal, breast and prostate cancer and colorectal adenoma. *International Journal of Cancer.* 2011 Mar 15;128(6):1414–24.

Huang Y, Nayak S. et al. Epigenetics in breast cancer: what's new? *Breast Cancer Research* 2011;13(6):225. Epub 2011 Nov 1.

Dumitrescu RG. Epigenetic markers of early tumor development. *Methods in Molecular Biology.* 2012;863:3–14. doi: 10.1007/978-1-61779-612-8_1.

Donovan M, Tiwary CM et al. Personal care products that contain estrogens or xenoestrogens may increase breast cancer risk. *Medical Hypotheses.* 2007;68(4):756–66. Epub 2006 Nov 28.

Wetherill YB, Fisher NL et al. Xenoestrogen action in prostate cancer: pleitropic effects dependent on androgen receptor status. *Cancer Research.* 2005 Jan 1;65(1):54–65.

Maffini MV, Rubin BS et al. Endocrine disruptors and reproductive health: the case of bisphenol-A. *Molecular and Cellular Endocrinology.* 2006 Jul 25;254-255:179–86. Epub 2006 Jun 15.

Section 5: Preventing Alzheimer's, Dementia And Age-Related Cognitive Decline

De la torre, JC. How do heart disease and stroke become risk factors for Alzheimer's disease? *Neurological Research.* 2006 Sep;28(6):637–44.

Whitmer, RA, Karter, AJ et al. Hypoglycemic episodes and risk of dementia in older patients with Type 2 diabetes mellitus. *Journal of the American Medical Association.* 2009;301(15):1565–1572. doi:10.1001/jama.2009.460.

Balion BJ, Gerard HC et al. Identification and localization of Chlamydia pneumoniae in the Alzheimer's brain. *Medical Microbiology and Immunology.* 1998 Jun;187(1):23–42.

Baudron CR, Letteneru L et al. Does helicobacter pylori infection increase incidence of dementia? *Journal of the American Geriatrics Society.* 2013;61(1):74–78.

Itzhaki RF, Wozniak MA. Herpes simplex virus type 1 in Alzheimer's disease: the enemy within. *Journal of Alzheimer's Disease.* 2008 May;13(4):393–405.

De la Monte SM, Neusner A et al. Epidemiological trends strongly suggest exposures as etiologic agents in the pathogenesis of sporadic Alzheimer's disease, diabetes mellitus, and non-alcoholic steatohepatitis. *Journal of Alzheimer's Disease.* 2009;17(3):519–29. doi: 10.3233/JAD-2009-1070.

Scarmeas N, Luchsinger JA et al. Physical activity, diet, and risk of Alzheimer disease. *Journal of the American Medical Association.* 2009 Aug 12;302(6):627–37. doi: 10.1001/jama.2009.1144.

Shrikant M, Kalpana P. The effect of curcumin (turmeric) on Alzheimer's disease: An overview. *Annals of Indian Academy of Neurology.* 2008 Jan–Mar; 11(1): 13–19. doi: 10.4103/0972-2327.40220.

Index

About the Author

After the terrorist bombings of September 11, 2001, Dr. John Salerno served as the medical director for the World Trade Center Landfill, a position that earned him a commendation from then-mayor Rudy Giuliani. In this capacity, he was charged with monitoring the health of the public workers assigned to manage the landfill where debris from the World Trade Center was transferred. It was on the site of this tragedy that Dr. Salerno began to formulate the Salerno Solution, a program for prevention and treatment of the chronic diseases of aging.

In addition to empowering his own patients with the strength to make healthy change, Dr. Salerno also provides specialized education to a large community of aspiring doctors at such prestigious schools as New York University physicians program, and New York College of Osteopathic Medicine where he lectures and teaches medical students on the importance of therapeutic wellness.

His exceptional ability to treat patients with chronic illnesses has placed him as:

- Cofounder of anti-aging clinics in New York City and Tokyo

- Chief medical officer behind the RenuLife anti-aging and dermatological clinic in Sao Paolo, Brazil

- International consultant for complementary medicine with seven affiliated centers in Tokyo, two in Brazil, and two in the U.S.

- His famous hands-on training for physicians and clinicians is sought after around the world

Dr. Salerno's desire for healing has led him to work alongside such holistic visionaries as:

- Dr. Robert C. Atkins (founder of the famous Atkins Diet)
- Suzanne Somers featured him in all of her bestselling books, *Ageless, Breakthrough* and *Knockout* for his extensive knowledge in the field of bioidentical hormone replacement therapy (BHRT).

Dr. Salerno developed and published *The Fight Fat with Fat Diet,* a three-step approach to nutrition based on:

1. Organic unprocessed foods

2. Low-carbohydrate intake

3. Targeted supplement protocols

Dr. Salerno is an author, lecturer, and media icon, whose work has been featured on:

- *Fox & Friends*
- *Fox News, Bloomberg*
- *Tokyo World News*
- WPIX
- *Sao Paulo International News*

In addition, he is a member of the:

- American Osteopathic Association
- American College for Advancement in Medicine
- American Medical Association

- American Academy of Anti-Aging Medicine
- International Society of Integrative Medicine
- Diplomat of the National Board of Osteopathic Medical Examiners
- Editorial Board Member of the International Society of Personalized Medicine Tokyo

A best-selling author, Dr. Salerno has been featured in:

- *The Huffington Post*
- *Personalized Medicine Universe*
- *Women's World*
- *Image Magazine*
- *New York Daily News* Online
- *Pur*
- *Belleza* magazine
- *Medical Spa and Resort Magazine*
- *Buena Vista News,* and other major media resources

Dr. Salerno also served as a clinical preceptor at the Yale University School of Medicine for three years, as Medical Director of St. Vincent's Immediate Health Care in Shelton, Connecticut, and lectured at the Vermont Family Practice Conference.

Stay in touch with Dr. Salerno through his website, www.salernocenter.com, where you can also access an exceptionally high-quality line of supplements that synchronize perfectly with his recommendations in this book.